Harnessing Full Value from the DoD Serum Repository and the Defense Medical Surveillance System

Melinda Moore, Elisa Eiseman, Gail Fisher,
Stuart S. Olmsted, Preethi R. Sama, John A. Zambrano

Prepared for the United States Army

ARROYO CENTER and RAND HEALTH

Center for Military Health Policy Research

The research described in this report was sponsored by the United States Army under Contract No. W74V8H-06-C-0001.

Library of Congress Cataloging-in-Publication Data

Harnessing full value from the DoD Serum Repository and the Defense Medical Surveillance System / Melinda Moore ... [et al.].
    p. cm.
 Includes bibliographical references.
 ISBN 978-0-8330-4910-0 (pbk. : alk. paper)
1. Medicine, Military—United States--Databases. 2. Serum—Collection and preservation—United States. I. Moore, Melinda.

UH223.H327 2010
616.9'8023—dc22

                                                        2010023629

The RAND Corporation is a nonprofit research organization providing objective analysis and effective solutions that address the challenges facing the public and private sectors around the world. RAND's publications do not necessarily reflect the opinions of its research clients and sponsors.

RAND® is a registered trademark.

Published 2010 by the RAND Corporation
1776 Main Street, P.O. Box 2138, Santa Monica, CA 90407-2138
1200 South Hayes Street, Arlington, VA 22202-5050
4570 Fifth Avenue, Suite 600, Pittsburgh, PA 15213-2665
RAND URL: http://www.rand.org/
To order RAND documents or to obtain additional information, contact
Distribution Services: Telephone: (310) 451-7002;
Fax: (310) 451-6915; Email: order@rand.org

Preface

For the past twenty years, the Department of Defense (DoD) has maintained a serum repository and associated database. Both of them have expanded in size, and in recent years they have been assigned additional mandates and requirements that extend beyond their original purpose, which was related to HIV testing, to serve deployment health surveillance and military force health protection more broadly. The Army's Center for Health Promotion and Preventive Medicine (CHPPM) serves as executive agent in managing the DoD Serum Repository (DoDSR) and Defense Medical Surveillance System (DMSS) on behalf of the entire department. As the mandate and value of these resources have grown, there has not been a commensurate systematic assessment of capabilities and untapped opportunities to better fulfill their missions, nor a consideration of how these might be better positioned to meet the needs of the military of the future. With these factors in mind, CHPPM commissioned this study, conducted from July 2006 to February 2008, to examine current requirements and capabilities, identify gaps, and suggest strategies to improve the capabilities of these resources to meet current and potential future needs in the areas of surveillance, outbreak investigation, research, and clinical support, particularly as these relate to influenza and other infectious disease threats.

This report should be of particular interest to health personnel in DoD, especially military health leaders and planners, those responsible for health surveillance across the services, medical providers, and health researchers. It should also be of interest to the Veterans Health Administration within the Department of Veterans Affairs, to the U.S. Congress, which has chartered within statute many of the functions of DoDSR and DMSS, and potentially to civilian health researchers.

This research was sponsored by the Army Medical Surveillance Activity under the Center for Health Promotion and Preventive Medicine. It was conducted within RAND Arroyo Center. The research was managed jointly by RAND Arroyo Center's Force Development and Technology Program, directed by Bruce Held, and the RAND Center for Military Health Policy Research, co-directed by Sue Hosek and Terri Tanielian. RAND Arroyo Center, part of the RAND Corporation, is the United States Army's federally funded research and development center for policy studies and analyses. The RAND Center for Military Health Policy Research is a joint endeavor of

RAND Arroyo Center and RAND Health. For more information on RAND Arroyo Center's Force Development and Technology Program, contact the Program Director, Bruce Held (telephone 310-393-0411, extension 7405, or by mail at RAND, 1776 Main Street, P.O. Box 2138, Santa Monica, CA 90407-2138).

The Project Unique Identification Code (PUIC) for the project that produced this document is CHPPM07260.

For more information on RAND Arroyo Center, contact the Director of Operations (telephone 310-393-0411, extension 6419; FAX 310-451-6952; email Marcy_Agmon@rand.org), or visit Arroyo's web site at http://www.rand.org/ard/.

Contents

Figures

Tables

Summary

The Department of Defense Serum Repository (DoDSR) and Defense Medical Surveillance System (DMSS) are longstanding and vital assets to U.S. Armed Forces medical surveillance. The repository contains over 43 million serial blood-derived serum specimens from over 10 million military applicants and active-duty and reserve service members over the course of their service careers; the DMSS database contains serial health data that can be linked to these specimens. Until late February 2008, the Army Medical Surveillance Activity (AMSA) managed both of these systems. On February 26, 2008, the Deputy Secretary of Defense signed a memorandum to create a new organization, the Armed Forces Health Surveillance Center (AFHSC), to oversee DoDSR and DMSS as well as the Global Emerging Infections Surveillance and Response System (GEIS).

In 2006, AMSA recognized that even though the DoDSR and DMSS had grown in response to evolving military health needs, their current and full potential use had not been systematically examined. Mindful of this, AMSA asked RAND to assess the DoDSR and DMSS to help identify ways for Army management to make them available to meet the health needs of the current and future military as fully as possible. The study was carried out between July 2006 and February 2008. The AFHSC now manages these important military assets. Updates since the creation of the AFHSC are outside the scope of this project and report. While RAND understands that some issues raised in this report may have been addressed already by AFHSC, we believe that the findings and recommendations in this report remain relevant.

The DoDSR and the associated DMSS database were originally designed for routine HIV screening purposes, but in recent years they have been assigned additional requirements related to deployment health and the prevention and control of diseases relevant to the military more broadly: force health protection. Over these years, the biological specimen used to fulfill new requirements has remained serum (the liquid component of blood), with serum specimens collected for all purposes archived in the DoDSR. With over 43 million specimens, the DoDSR is by far the largest serum repository in the country, perhaps the world. The associated DMSS database contains demographic and longitudinal service-related data and thus allows for analyses at a given period of time or over time; the ability to link such data with serum specimens creates a valuable surveillance resource for military health and even the broader civilian community, e.g., to the extent that detailed cross-sectional or longitudinal surveillance analyses in military populations reflect disease occurrences in the broader U.S. population.

This report focuses on the current and potential role of the DoDSR and associated DMSS database to support comprehensive health surveillance—referring to surveillance over the career lifetime of a service member and across all locations, epidemiological investigation, research, and clinical management. It describes current requirements and capabilities of both systems, presents findings and gaps, and assesses specific strategies to increase the capabilities of these vital surveillance resources to serve the needs of the U.S. Armed Forces today and into the future. We reviewed DoD policy, doctrine, and other published documents as well as published scientific literature, and we interviewed health experts inside and outside DoD to help identify and assess issues and their potential solutions. We also examined a number of other biological specimen repositories to glean insights potentially relevant to the DoDSR. We constructed a conceptual framework to help identify potential improvements to system elements and to organize the collection, analysis, and presentation of our data related to these potential improvements (Figure S.1).

Chapters One through Five frame the study (Chapter One), trace the evolution in requirements for the DoDSR and DMSS (Chapter Two), describe DoD's medical

Figure S.1
Conceptual Framework to Help Identify Potential Improvements to System Elements

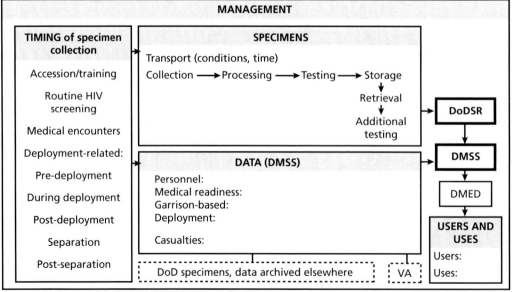

surveillance (Chapter Three), describe the current capabilities of AMSA, DoDSR, and DMSS (Chapter Four), and then examine other biological specimen repositories to glean insights potentially relevant to DoDSR (Chapter Five). Collectively, these establish the policy environment and baseline against which to assess future opportunities. Chapter Six then draws upon information related to current requirements and capabilities and our interviews to present findings and 26 potential improvement strategies organized according to our conceptual framework. The findings motivated potential improvement strategies addressing the following areas:

Management
- Mission (AMSA, DoDSR, DMSS)
- Organizational position of AMSA (through January 2008)
- Staffing
- Transparency for access to specimens
- Oversight of access to specimens
- Protection of human subjects
- Requirements for new repository storage space
- DMSS physical infrastructure and backup
- HIV and other screening

Timing of specimen collection
- Extending specimen collection beyond separation

Specimens
- Specimen processing and transport conditions
- Timing of specimen shipment to DoDSR
- Freeze-thaw cycles
- Size of aliquots to be released
- Screening beyond HIV
- Utility of serum and potential archiving of other blood fractions
- Storage conditions

Data
- Additional relevant data for DMSS
- Connection to other military biological specimen collections
- Behavioral risk factor data
- DMSS links to classified data
- Expanded access to DMSS data

Users and Uses
- Awareness of and demand for serum specimens and DMSS data
- Enhanced use for deployment health surveillance

- Expanded access to DoDSR specimens
- Enhanced use of serial specimens

Chapter Seven presents our recommendations, which reflect consolidated thematic packages of the strategies from Chapter Six, again organized based on our conceptual framework:

Management

1. Clarify and communicate the missions of DoDSR and DMSS both within and beyond DoD.

There is a mismatch between congressional direction for the use of the DoDSR and the DMSS data system as articulated in several enactments of the National Defense Authorization Act and the articulation of the mission and use of the DoDSR and DMSS by AMSA. Clear articulation by the new AFHSC and a common understanding across DoDSR and DMSS users of the full range of uses for these resources and their relative priority—including surveillance, epidemiologic investigation, clinical management, and research related to both infectious and noncommunicable diseases—should lead to their more efficient and robust use within DoD. Further, the mission of DoDSR and DMSS to collect specimens and data could also extend beyond DoD active and reserve populations to include continuation of data and specimen collection on a voluntary basis from separated service members followed in Military Treatment Facilities and/or the Veterans Health Administration system. To harness the full potential of the DoDSR and DMSS resources, AFHSC should establish the relative priority for the different uses and users of these resources and then make these explicit by communicating widely across DoD and into related research and epidemiologic communities if/as appropriate.

2. Empower, structure, and resource the organizational oversight of DoDSR and DMSS so that they can fulfill the full range of missions.

As we describe in the Authors' Note to our report (p. xxvii), DoD officially established the Armed Forces Health Surveillance Center within CHPPM in late February 2008. This organization is intended to encompass and integrate DoD-wide health surveillance. We hope that the AFHSC will be able to connect the various experts, contracts, and systems that are required not only for its primary surveillance mission but also for the full range of uses (primarily within the military but also extending to the civilian community) for the DoDSR and DMSS resources it manages through its executive agency function, including surveillance, epidemiologic investigation, clinical management, and research. Further, we hope that the chain of command and oversight for this organization will be such that it can receive guidance and resources from policymakers responsible for all of these functions, e.g., the Assistant Secretary of Defense (Health Affairs), Surgeons General, and Army Medical Research and Materiel

Command, in order to ensure proper alignment with current Military Health System strategy and resources and medical research and service health priorities as relevant to DoDSR and DMSS. The AFHSC should be configured and staffed to provide the support needed by all users, and especially those within the DoD, supporting execution of the designated missions for DoDSR and DMSS.

Data

3. Create an integrative data plan for comprehensive health surveillance.

Ideally, AFHSC should create an overarching and comprehensive data plan prescribing integration of all relevant heath surveillance data. Such a plan should address issues such as connectivity to occupational and environmental health surveillance systems, both within the garrison and in deployed settings, increasing data collection along the service member's period of service and beyond, and fully realizing policy efforts to facilitate access to surveillance and other data by the Department of Veterans Affairs (VA). Regarding DMSS specifically, several relevant military health datasets remain unconnected, thus limiting the full execution of AFHSC's surveillance mission and limiting the ability of DoD more broadly to take advantage of the full value offered by DMSS. The highest priorities for new data linkages into DMSS relate to deployment health, especially data derived from deployed settings. Current issues related to classified data systems also need to be overcome. We understand that relevant health surveillance data can possibly be made available to DMSS via the unclassified Theater Medical Data Store. For data that cannot be made available via this system, options for linking classified data into DMSS include time-delayed incorporation of declassified location data or near-real-time incorporation of classified data, which would require new secure communications capabilities that DMSS currently does not possess. Other relevant data linkages to consider are to existing DoD biological specimen archives such as isolates and original nasal swab specimens from the DoD Febrile Respiratory Illness surveillance system and pathology and necropsy specimens maintained by the Armed Forces Institute of Pathology in the National Pathology Repository. More robust linkages in both directions between DMSS and the VA health system should also be considered, to the extent that the mission of DoDSR and DMSS are expanded beyond strictly active-duty and reserve populations. Also, consideration should be given to whether and how behavioral risk factor data should be collected and fed into DMSS. Because there are many current data sources that might be tapped for deployment health surveillance, and there may be more in the future, the new AFHSC would be better positioned to fully execute its mission if it were included in the Military Health System information requirements process currently managed at the TRICARE Management Activity.

In addition to DMSS data content and management is the need for better protection of its physical infrastructure and the integrity of the data themselves, i.e., to resist physical or cyber threats to the DMSS database. In addition to assuring adequate housing of the data system, we recommend that strong consideration be given to systematic and frequent offsite backup and even parallel mirroring of the DMSS database, to assure its integrity in response to any threat that may arise, as occurred in late January 2008.

Specimens

4. Enhance the utility of specimens.

The DoDSR serum specimens continue to serve well their original purpose of HIV serosurveillance. However, as early as 1997, the DoD made a decision to continue using serum to meet new requirements related to biological specimens for deployment health surveillance. The sera permit examination of deployment-related exposures to and investigations of infectious agents; they are not particularly useful for time-sensitive environmental exposures for which biomarkers are only fleetingly present. And, as military health research becomes broader and more technologically sophisticated, the limitations of current serum specimens become more apparent: Researchers increasingly recognize the importance of genetic material for current and future research into a range of acute and chronic conditions. Serum specimens as presently stored in the DoDSR at –30°C do not reliably preserve genetic material. The best way to do this is to archive specimens derived from whole blood specimens, e.g., stored in liquid form or as dried blood spots, or storage of buffy coat fractions (see description in Chapter Five), in which the quantity of genetic material is substantially greater. Storage requirements for dried blood spots are modest and incrementally the easiest. Storage of both plasma and buffy coat at –80°C reflects current best industry practices for preservation of genetic material and other relevant blood-derived analytes. However, adoption of this alternative would mean costly new repository requirements for future specimens, i.e., walk-in freezers would not be possible for storage at –80°C. Nonetheless, the near-term expiration of the current repository lease and potential relocation provides a timely opportunity for military leadership to think carefully about the needs of the Military Health System into the future and determine whether new kinds of specimens should be archived, to better serve a broader range of mission areas for this valuable military resource.

5. Plan for the next repository facility.

Depending on decisions related to the strategies described in Chapter Six and the other recommendations here, DoD should begin already to define the requirements for the next repository, following expiration of the current lease in 2010. Factors to take into consideration include the time horizon for the next repository (e.g., 20 years or more), the annual rate of specimen acquisition (which would increase if specimens are to be collected from members following separation), the types of specimen to be archived (e.g., serum or plasma, buffy coat, whole blood in liquid form or as dried blood spots), and desired storage temperature (e.g., –30°C or –80°C). All of these influence the size and configuration of the future repository and hence the requirements for future repository space.

Users and Uses

6. Raise awareness of and expand access to DoDSR and DMSS.

The use of DoDSR and DMSS resources may be limited because of limited awareness across DoD. For example, military clinicians are apparently largely unaware of these resources in support of clinical management. Broad or targeted "educational campaigns" could be undertaken to raise awareness and use of DoDSR and DMSS. Access also may have been limited because of perceived lack of fully transparent criteria for release of specimens. A remedy for this could include development and dissemination of updated and transparent criteria and procedures for accessing DoDSR specimens and DMSS data. In terms of expanding use, the first priority should probably be for military health users within DoD, followed by more robust use by the VA. DoD should carefully consider whether and how to expand use to civilian researchers, while protecting individual privacy, the overall military health mission, and availability of remaining specimens as more users draw down the number of aliquots from a given specimen. Finally, efforts should be made to take better advantage of the longitudinal nature of the DoDSR inventory, e.g., through clarifying the legitimate use of DoDSR for research and sensitizing military health researchers to the availability of these serial specimens and linked data.

Conclusions

The goal of this study was to help identify opportunities to harness the full value of the DoDSR and DMSS assets—to make even better use of them in addressing military health needs now and into the future. Our analyses uncovered specific opportunities to better fulfill current requirements, especially to close gaps in the content and efficiency of medical surveillance. The largest gap relates to data from deployed settings, which figures prominently within the strategies we describe in the report and our recommendations. The DoDSR and DMSS serve their core surveillance mission; we have identified specific ways to position these resources to better serve the military of the future—planning now for changes that will permit a wider range of uses to improve not only surveillance but also clinical management and research in support of force health protection. Taken as a whole, our recommendations suggest that the DoDSR and DMSS will benefit from improved oversight and management to ensure they function within the strategic goals of the Military Health System, and have access to the needed data systems as well as other resources needed to fulfill the missions assigned to DoDSR and DMSS. Creation of the new AFHSC (after this study was completed) seems to be a good step in that direction, though detailed study of any new directions

AFHSC may be taking are beyond the scope of the present study. There are key decisions that need to be made at the Under Secretary of Defense level which will cascade across the recommendations we offer here, affecting the direction of the decisions as well as the magnitude of change.

AMSA was a responsible custodian for the DoDSR and DMSS, characterized by multiple interviewees as "national treasures" whose full potential has yet to be fully harnessed. Creation of the new AFHSC and relocation of the repository offer the opportunity to consider how the DoDSR and DMSS resources can be used to even greater advantage to support military health now and into the future. This study took a systematic approach to analysis of current characteristics and opportunities for improvement. Some of our recommendations are relatively easy, while others are more ambitious. Nonetheless, we feel that implementation of all of these recommendations will allow the AFHSC to better fulfill its current requirements, serve a broader range of legitimate mission areas, and position the DoDSR and DMSS resources for valuable service well into the future.

Acknowledgments

Many people gave generously of their time and expertise in support of this project. We thank all of the military personnel who provided extraordinarily useful information and insights about the current status and future potential of the DoD Serum Repository and Defense Medical Surveillance System, and also the civilian experts with whom we consulted with regard to their own programmatic assets and needs that might be relevant to these systems. CPT Remington Nevin, LTC Steven Tobler, and COL Robert DeFraites of the Armed Forces Health Surveillance Center greatly facilitated our work by providing both information and leads regarding sources of further information for our study. They also provided invaluable guidance from the inception of this project to its very end. We are indebted to our RAND colleagues Terri Tanielian and Sue Hosek for their careful and critical review of this work, and to Terri Tanielian, Sue Hosek, and Bruce Held for their supportive and helpful oversight. David Adamson and Kristin Leuschner provided thoughtful suggestions for the organization and presentation of the report, and Phil Kehres helped us prepare the final manuscript. We are grateful for comprehensive and thoughtful feedback on the final report from Dr. Patrick Kelley of the Institute of Medicine and Bernard Rostker of RAND. We hope that this report accurately captures the information and suggestions provided by all these individuals.

List of Acronyms

AFEB	Armed Forces Epidemiology Board
AFHSC	Armed Forces Health Surveillance Center
AFIOH	Air Force Institute for Operational Health
AFIP	Armed Forces Institute of Pathology
AHLTA	Armed Forces Health Longitudinal Technology Application
AMSA	Army Medical Surveillance Activity
ASD(HA)	Assistant Secretary of Defense (Health Affairs)
CDC	Centers for Disease Control and Prevention
CENTCOM	U.S. Central Command
CHPPM	Center for Health Promotion and Preventive Medicine
COCOM	Combatant Command
CONUS	Continental United States
DBS	Dried Blood Spots
DEDS	Directorate of Epidemiology and Disease Surveillance within CHPPM
DEERS	Defense Enrollment Eligibility Reporting System
DMED	Defense Medical Epidemiology Database
DMSS	Defense Medical Surveillance System
DNA	Deoxyribonucleic acid
DNBI	Disease and Non-Battle Injury
DoD	Department of Defense
DoDD	Department of Defense Directive
DoDI	Department of Defense Instruction
DoDSR	Department of Defense Serum Repository

ESSENCE	Electronic Surveillance System for the Early Notification of Community-Based Epidemics
FHP	Force Health Protection
FHP&R	Force Health Protection and Readiness (Division of ASD(HA))
FY	Fiscal Year
GEIS	Global Emerging Infections Surveillance and Response System
HHS	Department of Health and Human Services
HIV	Human Immunodeficiency Virus
ICD-9	International Classification of Diseases, Ninth Revision
IMR	Individual Medical Readiness
IQR	Interquartile Range
IRB	Institutional Review Board
JCS	Joint Chiefs of Staff
JMeWS	Joint Medical Workstation
JPTA	Joint Patient Tracking Application
MEPS	Military Entrance Processing Station
MILVAX	Military Vaccine Agency
MRMC	Medical Research and Materiel Command
MSMR	Medical Surveillance Monthly Report
MTF	Military Treatment Facility
NDAA	National Defense Authorization Act
NEHC	Naval Environmental Health Center
NHANES	National Health and Nutrition Examination Survey
NHLBI	National Heart, Lung, and Blood Institute
NHRC	Naval Health Research Center
NIPRNet	Non-Classified Internet Protocol Router Network (now known as Unclassified but Sensitive Internet Protocol Router Network)
OCONUS	Outside of Continental United States
OSD	Office of the Secretary of Defense
PDTS	Pharmacy Data Transaction Service
RBC	Red blood cells
RNA	Ribonucleic acid

SIPRNET	Secret Internet Protocol Router Network
SRSV	Secure Robotized Sample Vault
SSN	Social Security Number
TMDS	Theater Medical Data Store
TMIP	Theater Medical Information Program
VA	Department of Veterans Affairs
WBC	White blood cells
WRAIR	Walter Reed Army Institute of Research

Authors' Note

On February 26, 2008, the Deputy Secretary of Defense issued a memorandum officially establishing the Armed Forces Health Surveillance Center (AFHSC). Based on documents obtained by the RAND study team on February 28, this center had been in the planning stages since at least September 2005. In anticipation of its imminent formal establishment, the Army Surgeon General's office established a Provisional AFHSC in October 2007, combining two extant organizations: the Army Medical Surveillance Agency (AMSA) and the Global Emerging Infections Surveillance and Response System (GEIS). Both AMSA and GEIS are described in some detail in this report, and AMSA is in fact the focus of the report. Formalization of this new center occurred at the very end of this study. Because the new center combines two organizations, and because our study is in fact focused on AMSA, we have used the term AMSA throughout this report to refer to the portion of the new center that contains those activities performed by AMSA before the establishment of the AFHSC. Specifically, we are referring to the activities and responsibilities that involve management of the DoD Serum Repository and the Defense Medical Surveillance System.

CHAPTER ONE

Introduction

Protecting the health of military personnel is a strategic component of operational readiness. Force health protection is built upon a foundation of both individual medical care and public health services. In the public health area, the Department of Defense (DoD) provides preventive health services, monitors the health of its members using epidemiological surveillance, and, in the event of a disease outbreak, conducts disease investigation and response. Public health surveillance—i.e., the collection, analysis, and interpretation of health-related data and the dissemination of that information to monitor the health of a population and identify potential risks to health—is particularly important in deployed environments, where surveillance is used to inform operational readiness, track disease and injury, and permit examination of linkages between environmental exposures and health outcomes. Health data are critical to these activities and to ensuring the continuity of medical care over service members' careers.

Over the past 20 years, the DoD has collected blood specimens from both military members and applicants for service, and these specimens and related data have been stored in the DoD Serum Repository (DoDSR) and Defense Medical Surveillance System (DMSS), respectively. By the end of 2007, the repository contained over 43 million specimens taken from more than 10 million active-duty and reserve service members of the Army, Navy, Air Force, and Marines, and applicants to these services. The DMSS contains data linked to these specimens. Until late February 2008, the DoDSR and DMSS were both managed by the Army Medical Surveillance Activity (AMSA); since that time they now fall under management by the Armed Forces Health Surveillance Center (AFHSC).

Although routine collection of blood specimens was first mandated in 1985 to track the virus now known as HIV (with serum remaining after the tests retained in storage), the DoDSR has expanded in size and scope in recent years and is now intended to provide information about a number of deployment-related health issues and, more broadly, the identification, prevention, and control of disease associated with military service. DoDSR and DMSS can provide specimens and population-based information to the surveillance centers in other services as well as policymakers and researchers, and can also provide individual specimens and data to clinicians for medical management purposes. Since 1997, an important component of deployment health surveillance has been routine pre- and post-deployment health assessment and associated collection of blood specimens that are ultimately archived in the DoDSR for potential future testing.

However, while the mission and requirements of the DoDSR and DMSS have expanded, there has not been a commensurate systematic effort to assess how these resources are being managed and used, and whether there are opportunities for improvement in these areas. Therefore, in 2006 AMSA asked the RAND Corporation to undertake a systematic examination of DoDSR and DMSS to help identify ways to make these resources available to meet the current and future health needs of the military as fully as possible.

This report focuses on the current and potential role of the DoDSR and associated DMSS database to support comprehensive health surveillance, epidemiological investigation, research, and clinical management. It describes current requirements and capabilities of both systems, identifies issues and gaps, and assesses specific strategies to increase the capabilities of these vital surveillance resources to serve the needs of the U.S. Armed Forces today and into the future.

Purpose and Scope of RAND Study

The purpose of this study is to examine the current capabilities of the DoDSR and associated DMSS database in the areas of surveillance, epidemiologic investigation, research, and clinical support and to identify opportunities for improvement. To do this, we addressed five research questions:

- What are current requirements for collection and use of DoDSR specimens and DMSS data?
- What capabilities do the DoDSR and DMSS have to meet these requirements?
- How are the DoDSR and DMSS currently used?
- What are the gaps between current capabilities and current and potential future needs?
- What are strategies for improving capabilities to meet future needs?

We focused our examination of DoDSR and DMSS on considerations directly relevant to these systems and their military context:

- Blood and constituent components of potential use in surveillance, epidemiologic investigation, research, and clinical support;
- Infectious disease agents, as well as DNA and RNA, as the main target for testing from blood-derived specimens;
- Existing military data systems that could potentially be linked to DMSS; and
- Existing DoD policy, supporting programs, and legacy practices.

Methods

To answer the research questions, we:

- Reviewed DoD policy, doctrine, and other official documents;
- Reviewed peer-reviewed journal literature and written descriptions of relevant civilian repository programs;
- Compared the DoDSR to other selected military and civilian biological specimen repositories; and
- Conducted interviews (in person and via telephone) with persons whose experiences, responsibilities, and insights could inform potential improvements in the DoDSR and/or DMSS including DoD health leadership (six persons from OSD/Health Affairs); military surveillance centers from the Army (twelve persons), Navy (two persons) and Air Force (four persons); other military health experts (one from the Army's retrovirology laboratory, one from the Army Medical Examiner's office, three from the Uniformed Services University of the Health Sciences); and civilian health experts including nine from four different biospecimen repositories and one from the Department of Veterans Affairs); the questions in our semistructured interviews were organized based on the elements of the conceptual framework described below and asked about the experiences, perceptions, and suggestions the individuals had with regard to each of these elements.

We developed a conceptual framework (Figure 1.1) that organizes the system elements of the DoDSR and DMSS and depicts their logical relationship to one another. We used this framework to organize the collection of data from document review and interviews, guide identification of potential improvements for DoDSR and DMSS, and organize the analysis and presentation of our findings.

The system elements in our conceptual framework are as follows:

- **Management:** This domain includes the organization and staffing of AMSA (which until recently oversaw the DoDSR and DMSS and whose management responsibilities are now under the purview of the new AFHSC), the overall program direction and oversight, and management of the physical repository facility.
- **Timing of specimen collection:** Specimens are typically collected and archived from military service members. Figure 1.1 reflects a number of administrative milestones that already do, or could, trigger specimen collection over the term of a member's service.
- **Specimens:** Processes related to specimens include collection, processing, transport, initial testing, storage, retrieval, and additional testing.
- **Data:** This domain includes linkages of data into DMSS and access to the data.

Figure 1.1
Conceptual Framework to Help Identify Potential Improvements to System Elements

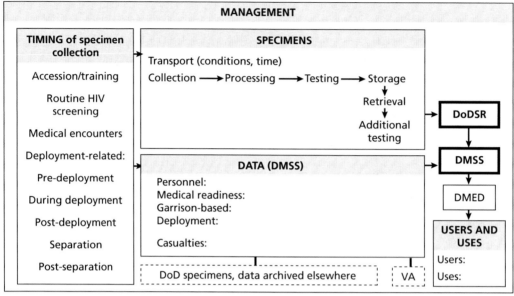

- **Users and uses:** This domain includes the range of military and nonmilitary users of DMSS data and/or DoDSR specimens, and the range of potential uses of these resources.

Organization of This Report

This report is organized as follows. Chapter Two describes the evolving requirements for DoDSR and DMSS, while Chapter Three describes selected military medical surveillance systems and organizations responsible for medical and broader health surveillance, to provide a context for the systems that currently are, or could be, linked to DMSS. Chapter Four describes the current capabilities of DoDSR and DMSS and of AMSA during the period of study (July 2006 to February 2008). Chapter Five examines other biological specimen repositories in order to seek insights that may be pertinent to decisions regarding DoDSR.

Chapter Six then uses the conceptual framework described above as the basis for presenting our findings and potential strategies to close gaps between requirements and current capabilities and to increase the capabilities of DoDSR and DMSS to meet new needs into the future. Chapter Seven concludes with a description of six overarching recommendations derived from our analyses.

CHAPTER TWO

Evolution of DoDSR and DMSS Requirements

In order to evaluate how well the DoDSR and DMSS are able to meet current and future requirements, we need first to understand what those requirements are and how they have evolved since the DoDSR was first created in 1985. We begin by discussing the current mission of the DoDSR and DMSS and the way in which the requirements have evolved over time. Figure 2.1 depicts the main highlights of this evolution, and Appendix A presents a more detailed summary of the requirements as they have evolved. We also discuss aspects of DoD's vision for the repository and ways in which its role was intended to develop.

Evolving Mission and Uses of the DoDSR

The current mission of the DoDSR is to provide support for the identification, prevention, and control of disease related to military service (DoDD 6490.02E). The mission of the DMSS is to serve as a tri-service medical surveillance system.

The uses of the repository have shifted, however. The DoDSR was initially conceived as a resource derived from routine HIV screening. It subsequently was defined also as a resource for deployment health surveillance, and later for the even broader purpose of identifying, preventing, and controlling disease associated with all military service, especially infectious and other diseases for which biomarkers can be found in stored specimens.

We describe highlights from this evolution in the following subsections. Figure 2.1 gives an overview of the main steps in the evolution.

Origins in HIV Screening Program

The serum collection currently maintained in the DoDSR and managed by AMSA until late February 2008 started in 1985 as part of the Army's HTLV-III screening program (ASD(HA), 1985), which began in response to the spread of a new human virus subsequently known as the human immunodeficiency virus (HIV). DoD instituted mandatory collection of blood specimens for screening of all civilian applicants going through Military Entrance Processing Stations (MEPS). Actual collection and storage

Figure 2.1
Evolution of DoDSR, DMSS, and Organizational Requirements

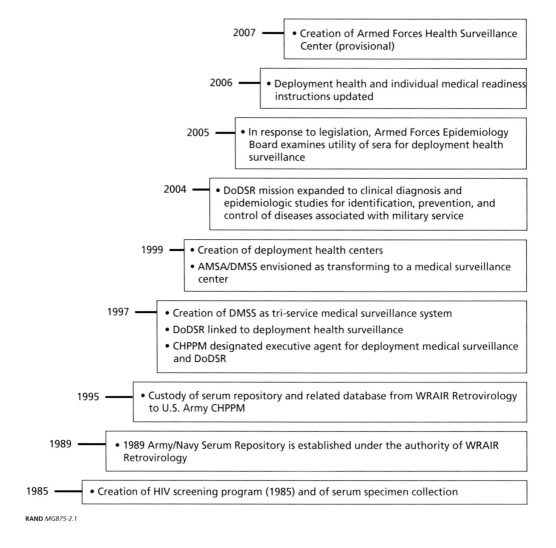

2007 — • Creation of Armed Forces Health Surveillance Center (provisional)

2006 — • Deployment health and individual medical readiness instructions updated

2005 — • In response to legislation, Armed Forces Epidemiology Board examines utility of sera for deployment health surveillance

2004 — • DoDSR mission expanded to clinical diagnosis and epidemiologic studies for identification, prevention, and control of diseases associated with military service

1999 — • Creation of deployment health centers
• AMSA/DMSS envisioned as transforming to a medical surveillance center

1997 — • Creation of DMSS as tri-service medical surveillance system
• DoDSR linked to deployment health surveillance
• CHPPM designated executive agent for deployment medical surveillance and DoDSR

1995 — • Custody of serum repository and related database from WRAIR Retrovirology to U.S. Army CHPPM

1989 — • 1989 Army/Navy Serum Repository is established under the authority of WRAIR Retrovirology

1985 — • Creation of HIV screening program (1985) and of serum specimen collection

RAND *MG875-2.1*

of remnant serum occurred as part of contracts between DoD and commercial testing laboratories in which all nonreactive serologic specimens were ordered to remain in frozen storage for the duration of the contract. Although these disparate collections of serum, which would ultimately seed the DoDSR inventory, were stored by the DoD contractors, a specified purpose for their future use had not been officially articulated. In 1989, a maintenance and management contract was awarded to McKesson to begin consolidating and storing in a single facility the serum specimens that were stored by testing contractors, who had been conducting HIV screening for the DoD since 1985.

Under the authority of the Walter Reed Army Institute of Research (WRAIR) Division of Retrovirology, this contract gave way to the establishment of the Army/Navy Serum Repository, the predecessor to the DoDSR. By 1990, the contractor processing the HIV specimens had collected and stored over six million serum specimens.

The first officially articulated purpose of the repository was documented in a 1991 Army request for proposals to create and maintain the Walter Reed Army Serum Bank Repository: "Sera repository operations are required for retrospective studies in support of current and future retroviral research efforts . . . Analysis of these sera will be very important." Walter Reed's Division of Retrovirology would require as-needed specimen retrieval up to about 5,000 per year.

By 1996, the repository had collected and stored over 17 million serum specimens from Army and Navy civilian applicants as well as from active component service members (Institute of Medicine, 1996). Together with the linked medical information stored in the U.S. Army HIV Data System, the military had developed a rich resource for conducting robust retrospective studies.

Along with the creation of the serum repository, the Army created a data center in 1986 within the WRAIR Division of Preventive Medicine to support HIV-related screening, care, and research activities (Rubertone and Brundage, 2002). In 1995 the system was transferred to the Army's Center for Health Promotion and Preventive Medicine (CHPPM) and called the Army Medical Surveillance System

Emergence of Deployment Health Surveillance Requirements

Later in the 1990s, the serum repository was assigned an additional mission related to deployment health, and AMSA was designated as executive agent responsible for management of the repository and associated data system on behalf of DoD. Many service members returning from the first Gulf War reported illnesses of unknown origin, and many questioned the DoD's commitment to providing health care for military members and veterans. The issues were so serious that in the decade after the war, DoD sought to determine not only the etiology of the illnesses and appropriate treatments, but also sought to establish systems that would assure capture of adequate health data in future deployments. This was important because the medical records of deployed Gulf War service members were not adequate either to substantiate or refute the exposures being reported. Public concern was so great that even as late as 2000, the Institute of Medicine published a report criticizing the DoD for not adequately addressing the concerns that had been raised and urging DoD to take "immediate action" to repair the data deficiencies in the medical records of service members (Institute of Medicine, 2000).

In response to the concerns over what became known as "Gulf War Illness," in 1997 Congress mandated that DoD conduct comprehensive health surveillance on service members who deploy overseas (Public Law 105-85, 1997). In particular, the law required DoD to collect blood specimens before and after military deployments. It also stipulated that DoD maintain a central archive of records and make them accessible across DoD.

Nearly simultaneously, DoD issued new policy related to joint medical surveillance (DoDD 6490.2 and DoDI 6490.3). These policy issuances designated CHPPM as executive agent for deployment medical surveillance and for maintenance of a DoD-wide serum repository whose purpose was "medical surveillance for clinical diagnosis and epidemiologic studies. The repository shall be used exclusively for the identification, prevention and control of diseases associated with operational deployments of military personnel" (DoDD 6490.2, para D7). CHPPM was also directed to "maintain a medical surveillance system to integrate, analyze, and report data from multiple sources relevant to the health and readiness of military personnel" (DoDI 6490.3, para E7); the services, components, and combatant commands (COCOMs) were mandated to report data to CHPPM.

It is important to note that the serum repository, which had originally been established in response to then-available technology for HIV screening, was essentially expanded to also serve as a deployment health surveillance tool, with serum remaining the biological specimen used to meet this new requirement. It is also important to note that the 1997 policy appears to limit the use of the serum repository to deployment-related health. These points had many implications, which we will examine in some detail later in this report.

Also in 1997, the Assistant Secretary of Defense (Health Affairs) (ASD(HA)) called for the creation of a tri-service medical surveillance system; this became the DMSS at CHPPM.[1] Also at this same time, the Army's Medical Surveillance System changed its name to be the DMSS and was moved from being managed directly by CHPPM to being managed by AMSA, a subordinate agency of CHPPM (Rubertone and Brundage, 2002).

Vision for All-Theater Medical Surveillance and Data Collection. In 1998, the ASD(HA) issued a policy memorandum which established that a pre- and post-deployment blood specimen collection (mandated by the National Defense Authorization Act (NDAA) of FY98) could be met by routine participation in the HIV screening program, as long as the pre-deployment specimen was collected within 12 months of the start of the deployment (ASD(HA), October 6, 1998).

In further response to the health problems experienced by the veterans of the first Gulf War, Congress passed the NDAA for FY99 (Public Law 105-261, 1998), which authorized the Secretary of Defense to establish a center for deployment health in which longitudinal health data would be collected and studied in order to assess the effect of deployment on service members (section 743).

---

[1]   We were unable to find the source document, but were able to find reference to it in an ASD(HA) memorandum from September 30, 1999, which we describe in more detail later in this report.

Because of this legislation, the ASD(HA) issued a key policy memorandum in 1999 that established two centers for deployment health—the Deployment Health Clinical Center within the Walter Reed Army Medical Center and the Deployment Health Research Center within the Naval Health Research Center—and specified that the DMSS would serve as the "comprehensive, longitudinal, relational, epidemiology database" for the study of deployment-related health (see Figure 2.1). This memorandum explicitly calls for "all theater medical surveillance and treatment data collected by the Services, Unified and Specified Commands and individual commands . . . (to be) forwarded to the DMSS." Finally, it stipulates that the "TRICARE Management Activity will provide unrestricted access to applicable Military Health System data and support the DMSS . . . as appropriate" (ASD(HA), September 30, 1999, para 6). The same memorandum provides a concept for changing the DMSS into a "DoD Medical Surveillance Agency" that would function as the DoD's deployment health surveillance center (Concept of Operations attachment).

The concept for the future of DMSS was that it would provide access to deployment-related health data and allow for DoD-wide surveillance and research. CHPPM was designated as the DoD repository for all theater medical surveillance data, as described above, and AMSA was described as "the sole link between the DoD Serum Repository and other databases" (ASD(HA), 1999). And finally, DMSS was directed to provide remote access to personnel and health surveillance data to the Naval Health Research Center (NHRC) and other related service surveillance organizations. As we describe in later chapters of this report, not all the provisions of this memorandum were executed.

Therefore, by the end of FY99, DoD had established a deployment-related health surveillance system with the goal of determining the health effects of deployment; established three deployment health centers, each with a distinct deployment-health mission (clinical, research, surveillance); and established a data system in order to assess deployment-related health data. Most of the major groundwork for deployment health surveillance was begun.

Effect of the Global War on Terror. The Global War on Terror created new demands related to medical surveillance and deployment health surveillance, and these played out in the modifications to the required deployment health assessment forms (DD Forms 2795 and 2796), in the expansion of the surveillance program to cover certain reserve component populations, and in development of quality assurance programs. Importantly, in 2001, ASD(HA) issued a policy memorandum that applied all deployment-related health assessment requirements and specimen collection requirements to the reserve component service members who were activated for 30 days or more. This memorandum required that all pre- and post-deployment health assessment forms (DD Forms 2795 and 2796, respectively) be sent to AMSA and stipulated the content of the forms by providing examples within the memorandum which were mandated across services. Further policy issuances updated procedures for deployment health surveillance and readiness (JCS, 2002), enhanced post-deployment assessments (USD(P&R), 2003), and new requirements for the electronic transmission and capture of pre- and post-deployment health assessment forms (ASD(HA), 2004).

Broadening of Mission Beyond Deployment Health

The mission and requirements for DoDSR expanded further beginning in 2004, when the use of the repository was broadened beyond exclusive use for deployment-related health to encompass all uses for the prevention and control of diseases associated with military service. This began when DoD issued a major policy document in 2004 describing the overarching guidelines and goals for force health protection within the Military Health System (DoDD 6200.04). This document lays out requirements for annual health assessments, as well as annual assessments of individual medical readiness. Individual medical readiness standards are applied to each individual service member to ensure their ability to deploy worldwide, and are further described in Chapter Three.

Less than two weeks later, DoD issued new policy on Comprehensive Health Surveillance (DoDD 6490.02E), updating the 1997 issuance on joint medical surveillance (see Figure 2.1). The 2004 policy document described a broader mission for the repository:

> 4.12 There shall be a Department of Defense Serum Repository for medical surveillance for clinical diagnosis and epidemiologic studies. The repository shall be used for the identification, prevention and control of disease associated with military service.

The 2004 comprehensive health surveillance issuance establishes DoD policy to conduct health surveillance across service members' careers, in all duty locations and across the full spectrum of activities encountered within the military. It requires daily review of battle injuries and disease and non-battle injuries in order to detect any health threats; it directs biological monitoring as required; and it directs that tri-service reportable medical events be reported electronically, although neither the reporting system nor the reporting destination is specified. That is, the policy directs collection of such data but does not explicitly link this to DMSS. The comprehensive health surveillance issuance also requires the synchronization of data between medical and personnel systems and directs that health surveillance data be transferred to the Department of Veterans Affairs once a service member separates from the service.

In sum, by 2004, the mission and requirements related to DoDSR had evolved beyond HIV screening and deployment health surveillance to also include a broader range of purposes: medical surveillance, clinical diagnoses, and epidemiologic studies for diseases associated with military service, i.e., not strictly limited to deployment health surveillance.

Growing Concern About DoD's Ability to Track and Assess Deployment Health Data

By 2005, the Global War on Terror was four years underway and record numbers of reserve component deployments supplemented high levels of active component deployments. Congress in 2005 again addressed the issue of deployment health surveillance. The NDAA of FY05 indicated growing congressional concern with the DoD's ability to track and assess deployment health data, especially data from theater, given the high levels of deployments and complex nature of the contingencies in Iraq and Afghanistan. In particular, the NDAA for 2005 contained several requirements:

- The Secretary of Defense was to ensure interim standards that blood specimens needed for the pre-deployment examination of a service member be drawn no later than 120 days prior to the date of the deployment, and that the post-deployment specimens be drawn no later than 30 days after the conclusion of the deployment (section 734).
- DoD was to maintain a medical record of all care provided to service members in theater as part of a complete health record.
- Medical tracking and health surveillance in-theater systems were to be evaluated, with a report due back to Congress within a year. The evaluation was to establish "the efficacy of health surveillance as a means of detecting (i) any health problems (including mental health conditions) of members of the Armed Forces . . . ; and (ii) exposures of assessed members to environmental hazards that potentially lead to future health problems" (para B). Further, Congress required the evaluation to address how the data system could support future research on health issues, to make recommendations for changes to medical tracking and health surveillance systems, and to provide a summary of scientific literature on blood sampling procedures used for detecting and identifying exposures (paras C–E). Congress also asked DoD to determine in this same evaluation whether a need existed for "changes to regulations and standards for drawing blood specimens for effective tracking and health surveillance of the medical conditions of personnel before deployment, upon the end of deployment, and for a follow up period of appropriate length" (para F).
- DoD was to prescribe a policy on the collection and dissemination of in-theater individual personnel locations (section 734, para D).
- DoD was to review and revise the classification levels of data for the use of monitoring and assessing the health tracking and surveillance data in order to make the data more useful (section 735).

While deployment health surveillance and medical surveillance, epidemiology and clinical support are not mutually exclusive, it was clear that Congress's interest lay in assuring that the DoDSR and DMSS met all key needs as a deployment health surveillance tool. Yet neither Congress nor DoD explicitly specified DMSS as the destination for theater medical surveillance data.

Potential Need for Changes in the Process of Drawing Blood Samples. In addition, the NDAA required the DoD to examine the need for any changes related to the process of drawing blood specimens for effective deployment health surveillance. In order to conduct the evaluation required by Congress, the ASD(HA) requested a study from the Armed Forces Epidemiology Board (ASD(HA), 2005), posing three questions:

- Is there a sound basis for the continued routine collection of sera pre- and post-deployment for clinical care reasons, public health surveillance, or research purposes in order to examine the effects of deployment on health?
- Should any other biological specimens be collected for clinical care reasons, public health surveillance, or research purposes?
- Are there were any valid reasons to change the time frames of specimens of collected biological specimens either pre- or post-deployment for clinical care reasons, public health surveillance, or research purposes?

The study reached four conclusions (Armed Forces Epidemiology Board, 2005). First, it concluded that there were medically valid reasons to continue the collection of serum specimens for all purposes. Next, the study concluded that there is utility in collecting baseline and periodic blood specimens consisting of serum and white blood cells. Going further, the study suggested that DoD should formalize in rules and procedures and make more clear the accessibility of the repository, to ensure wide access, and also that an oversight panel be created to govern access. Finally, the study concluded that sampling of the entire deploying military force, as opposed to a smaller sample of the deploying population, was also appropriate for the purposes of deployment health surveillance, and that the one-year pre-deployment and 30-day post-deployment collection windows were appropriate.

As provided for in the NDAA FY05, the ASD(HA) changed the legislated interim standards for pre- and post-deployment serum collection per the recommendations of the Armed Forces Epidemiology Board, allowing pre-deployment serum specimens to be collected within 365 days of deployment under routine HIV sampling, unless some reason would indicate a more proximate collection, and post-deployment serum collection within 30 days after arrival at a demobilization site or home station or in-patient medical treatment facility in the case of evacuees (ASD(HA), 2006).

Establishment of Policy on Individual Medical Readiness. As the conflict in Iraq changed from a major combat operation to a counterinsurgency operation, veterans began to return to the United States with blast injuries from improvised explosive devices. Injuries involving extremities were seen more often, as were blast injuries and psychological traumas that were manifesting themselves months after the deployment in cognitive and mental health problems. In March 2005, the ASD(HA) issued a policy memorandum that required a new post-deployment health reassessment form that was to be completed between three and six months following a deployment. Although the new form was designed to elicit a service member's concern about physical health, its focus was on self-perceived cognitive and psychological health issues. The form was based on the pre- and post-deployment health assessment forms and was to be ultimately funneled to AMSA for storage in DMSS and inclusion in required analyses of deployment health assessments.

By 2006, the manpower-intensive counterinsurgency efforts in Iraq and Afghanistan demanded new sources of U.S. troops, with Navy personnel being used on the ground in Iraq, for example. Because of the relatively large demand on both active and reserve service members for ground operations, DoD issued new policy on individual medical readiness establishing six baseline readiness standards across all services (DoDI 6025.19). The medical readiness standards for deployment for individuals are: (1) a current periodic health assessment (every 12 months), (2) the absence of deployment-limiting medical conditions, (3) dental readiness to specified standards, (4) immunization standards germane to the theater of operation, (5) current medical readiness laboratory tests, and (6) possession of appropriate individual medical equipment. These new standards eased the confusion that arose from competing standards across services, while also creating a sort of baseline for surveillance of medical readiness across DoD (see Figure 2.1).

In 2006 DoD updated its 1997 deployment health policy to specify policies and procedures for daily monitoring of disease and non-battle injury rates during deployments (the diseases and injuries incurred during a deployment but not from combat), address occupational and environmental health risk, require documentation of occupational and environmental health exposures, and require a record of daily location of personnel (DoDI 6490.03). This issuance also requires that deployment health data be collected, transmitted, and maintained electronically, rather than on paper as had been previously practiced, although the systems were not specified, i.e., DMSS was never mentioned as the destination for such deployment health surveillance data.

The updated 2006 deployment health policy responded to the outstanding requirement from the NDAA FY05 for more complete and accurate individual location data by directing the Deputy Under Secretary of Defense for Program Integration to ensure that the current manpower data center receive once-daily deployment location records at the Secret level and below. This allows linkages between exposures and patient encounter data. The services are tasked within this instruction to develop a data collection system that would record the location data of all deployed individuals. The services are further tasked to ensure post-deployment health assessment and reassessment forms are submitted to DMSS, and to conduct occupational and environmental health surveillance (section 5). The COCOMs are tasked to coordinate occupational and environmental and medical surveillance, and to provide timely reporting of disease and non-battle injuries, battle injuries, and other medical events (section 5).

The updated 2006 deployment health policy reiterates the maintenance of DMSS and DoDSR by AMSA, and the timelines for pre- and post-deployment serum sampling and process. It tasks AMSA with providing individual-level and aggregated data from the pre- and post-deployment health assessment forms as well as the reassessment form. It also directs AMSA to integrate tri-service reportable medical events data from across the services and make such data available to the services for further analyses and reporting. It further directs the Army to maintain and provide analyses from the occupational and environmental health data system. Yet, while DMSS is explicitly mentioned in the context of ongoing pre- and post-deployment health assessment forms, there is no mention that directs theater surveillance data be sent or ultimately linked into DMSS.

Chapter Highlights

There are several points to be emphasized from this discussion of requirements to inform the future of DoD's medical and deployment health surveillance, the serum repository, and DMSS.

- In terms of current missions:
  - The policy-directed mission for AMSA was—and for AFHSC now includes—to manage the DoDSR and DMSS and to act as the organization carrying out the Secretary of the Army's executive agency responsibility for DoD-wide deployment medical surveillance;
  - The current policy-directed mission of the DoDSR is to provide support for the identification, prevention and control of disease related to military service;
  - The current policy-directed mission of the DMSS is to act as a tri-service medical surveillance system that is to transform to a medical surveillance center, share data across services with related surveillance agencies, connect to all relevant personnel and medical systems, and receive all theater medical data. Yet no policy specifies that theater medical surveillance data be transmitted to DMSS.

- The use of the repository has grown since its inception in 1985. Initially a resource derived from routine HIV screening, it subsequently became a resource for deployment health surveillance, and later as a resource for the broader purpose of identification, prevention, and control of disease associated with all military service, for both the reserve and active components.

- As early as 1997, DoD determined that it would continue to store the sera that had already been collected and also continue to use serum specimens to fulfill new deployment health surveillance requirements. Pursuant to legislation in 2005, the ASD(HA) requested an evaluation of the soundness of the continued use of sera for surveillance and for clinical care purposes as well as research. The Armed Forces Epidemiology Board conducted the evaluation and reported that there was utility in continuing this practice, but suggested that archiving of an additional blood fraction—white blood cells—might also be appropriate in order to preserve genetic material for testing now and into the future. As we discuss later in this report, with the technological advances presenting new opportunities for health surveillance, the benefits of storing whole blood, or other blood fractions, may now outweigh the convenience of continuing to rely solely upon serum as the biological specimen used to meet deployment health surveillance requirements now and into the future.

- In 1997 the ASD(HA) envisioned DMSS as a tri-service medical surveillance data system that would be connected to health data collections in a theater of operation. ASD(HA) further suggested that DMSS would migrate toward a "DoD Medical Surveillance Agency" that would function as the DoD's deployment health surveillance center. As we discuss later in our report, this suggestion has never been realized. Data collected from theater systems have not been fed into DMSS, but instead these data are being analyzed by an agency within ASD(HA). Further, the collection of individual location data has been addressed both by Congress and DoD, yet as we discuss later, these data are still elusive. In fact, the connection of the DMSS system to relevant and timely data systems is a significant issue that can be addressed by DoD, since there appears to be regulatory guidance available and the data systems themselves are evolving to make such connections more feasible.

In this chapter we have discussed the statutory and DoD policy directives relating to AMSA, the DoDSR, and DMSS. In the next chapter we will describe selected DoD medical surveillance systems and organizations.

CHAPTER THREE

Department of Defense Medical Surveillance

We now discuss DoD surveillance systems. Understanding relevant medical surveillance activities helps place the role of DoDSR and DMSS into context. The summaries of relevant surveillance components and activities also set the stage for potential strategies to improve the capabilities of DoDSR and DMSS by leveraging, integrating, or streamlining existing DoD activities and resources.

DoD distinguishes between "medical surveillance" and "health surveillance." Medical surveillance involves the collection, management, and analysis of health and medical information, including biological specimens, from members of all services stationed in both garrison and deployed environments in the United States and around the globe. Health surveillance is broader: it includes medical surveillance as well as occupational and environmental health surveillance. The military operational tempo since 2001 has led to updates in DoD policy related to deployment health, including deployment health surveillance.

Guided by department policy, the services carry out routine public health surveillance activities such as HIV testing (DoDD 6485.1), notifiable disease reporting (ASD(HA), November 9, 1998), and disease and non-battle injury reporting (DoDI 6490.03). Independently, services support more specialized public health programs based on the needs of their member population and operations. Specific service components have been designated to support DoD-wide public health program elements.

Our focus in this chapter is on medical surveillance within the broader context of health surveillance in DoD. The goal is to describe the scope of these activities across DoD along with the current systems executing them. We discuss selected medical surveillance systems and the organizational components responsible for medical and broader military health surveillance. We begin with a discussion of relevant definitions and principles established by DoD policy, then highlight relevant surveillance systems, and finally discuss key service agencies that conduct military health surveillance.

Key Definitions

Department of Defense policy has defined different kinds of military health surveillance, based on the source, content, and scope of the data. These definitions begin to establish the context for the role of DoDSR and DMSS. The following definitions are taken from DoDD 6490.02E, with key distinctions across definitions highlighted:

(3.1) Comprehensive Military Health Surveillance.

Health surveillance conducted throughout **Service members' military careers, across all duty locations, and encompassing risk, intervention, and outcome data.** Such surveillance is essential to the evaluation, planning, and implementation of public health practice and prevention and must be closely integrated with the timely dissemination of information to those who can act upon it.

(3.2) Health Surveillance.

The regular or repeated collection, analysis, and interpretation of health-related data and the dissemination of information to monitor the health of a population and to identify potential risks to health, thereby enabling timely interventions to prevent, treat, or control disease and injury. It includes occupational and environmental health surveillance and medical surveillance.

(3.3) Medical Surveillance.

The ongoing, systematic collection, analysis, and interpretation of **data derived from instances of medical care or medical evaluation,** and the reporting of population-based information for characterizing and countering threats to a population's health, well-being, and performance.

(3.4) Occupational and Environmental Health Surveillance.

The regular or repeated collection, analysis, archiving, interpretation, and dissemination of **occupational and environmental health related data** for monitoring the health of, or potential health hazard impact on, a population and individual personnel, and for intervening in a timely manner to prevent, treat, or control the occurrence of disease or injury when determined necessary.

Medical Surveillance Systems Across DoD

This section describes a range of DoD's medical surveillance systems and activities. Not surprisingly, data systems are stovepiped within services. Moreover, as noted in Chapter Two, the regulatory context for deployment health has developed separately from the garrison, or nondeployment, context. Data collection systems have likewise developed within those two general contexts, as we describe below.

Table 3.1
Summary of Elements Within Selected Military Medical Surveillance Systems

System	Specimens	Data	Reports	Data in DMSS?
HIV screening	Serum (DoDSR)	Date, service, SSN	HIV trends	Yes
Deployment health assessment	None	DD Forms 2795, 2796, 2900	Monthly MSMR reports	Yes
Reportable medical events	None	70 specified diseases and conditions	Daily reports monitored by services	Garrison: Yes Deployed: No
Mortality	None (for surveillance)	Cause-specific mortality, near real-time	Weekly casualty reports	No (discontinued in 2003)
Disease and nonbattle injury	None	Inpatient and outpatient, ICD-9 codes, individual	Aggregate data reports, through JMeWS	No
Individual medical readiness	(HIV, forensic DNA)	Six standard indicators[a]	Visibility at service level; reported to OSD	Immunizations, HIV: Yes Others: No

[a] These indicators were developed for purposes of ensuring medical readiness for deployment, but are included here because some are potentially relevant for surveillance purposes.

We identified relevant systems that collect, analyze, and report medical data used to monitor the health of service members and prevent, treat, or control disease and injury. For each surveillance system, we describe the main purpose and relevant doctrine and also present brief descriptions of the data collected in support of the surveillance mission, reports generated by the systems, and whether or not these data are sent to DMSS. A high-level summary of the information discussed in this chapter is provided in Table 3.1. A detailed description of the capabilities of DoDSR and DMSS is provided in Chapter Four.

Human Immunodeficiency Virus-1 (HIV-1)

DoDD 6485.1, issued in 1992, assigns responsibility to the Secretary of each Military Department to establish policies and programs for the identification, surveillance, education, and administration of personnel infected with HIV-1. At present, the interval for periodic screening of personnel through the collection and testing of serum specimens is not to exceed 24 months.

Specimens collected by the Army and Navy are tested and processed by ViroMed, a contract laboratory. Specimens drawn for Air Force personnel are tested and processed by the Air Force Institute for Operational Health (AFIOH). Specimens collected from all services are shipped to DoDSR for frozen storage.

Deployment-Related Health Assessments

Pre- and Post-Deployment and Health Assessment Forms, DD Forms 2795 and 2796, and associated blood specimens are the basis for the deployment health surveillance carried out previously by AMSA and now by AFHSC. The forms are completed by all military personnel before and after serving in major overseas deployments in compliance with DoD Instruction 6490.03, "Deployment Health," August 2006. All deployment-related health assessment forms are submitted electronically to DMSS and permanently archived. A post-deployment health reassessment requirement was added in 2005, instituting collection of health information and a medical review of service members 3–6 months after returning from deployment. The program uses DD Form 2900 to collect information on health concerns, with particular emphasis on mental health; the latest version of the form is dated January 2008.

The pre-deployment process generally involves self-disclosure by a service member of any recent health events, medicines being taken, and any health concerns. Once the form is completed, medical personnel will review the form and if needed interview the service member to determine fitness for deployment or if the service member needs any treatment to prepare for deployment. The post-deployment assessment process starts with the completion of the form by a service member. When a concern is noted on the form or the service member screens positively for potential mental or physical health issues, that member is immediately seen by medical personnel who will determine whether referral to a medical provider for further attention is needed. The post-deployment reassessment process is similar to the post-deployment process, but is focused on capturing cognitive and mental health problems, which typically appear in the three- to six-month window following return from a deployment. Again, should a service member screen positive or indicate health concerns in their reassessment, he or she will be seen by medical personnel and referred as appropriate.

The deployment health assessment forms are intended to describe the service members' perceptions of their own health, health exposures, psychological problems, and health-related concerns, the post-deployment health assessment and reassessment forms in particular. However, some limitations exist in these forms, restricting their use in robust population-level analysis. Information intended to describe in-theater health and exposure concerns is captured post-deployment through self-report, introducing the opportunity for recall bias and limited specificity. The questions differ between pre- and post-deployment forms, and different versions of the forms have been used over the years. In addition, the response categories to questions addressing health and exposure concerns are broad and restricted to self-report. Analyses have been conducted using these data: the Medical Surveillance Monthly Report (MSMR) publishes monthly tabulations of self-assessed health status, including mental health referrals. The forms are currently undergoing validation by the Military Health System.

Reportable Medical Events Surveillance

There are two separate systems for reportable medical event surveillance. In a deployment setting, the Joint Staff sets the tri-service surveillance reporting requirements for deployments, which currently include 70 types of medical events to which others can be added by COCOMs and joint task forces as needed (JCS, 2007). Theater-based information is reported through the Joint Medical Workstation (JMeWS).

For the garrison setting, the services participate in a Joint Preventive Medicine Policy Group which establishes the list of required medical events that must be reported. Reporting requirements are established under the authority of the ASD(HA) and were published previously by AMSA (ASD(HA), November 6, 1998). In garrison, current reporting of selected medical events relies on a passive approach based on identification and coding by physicians during medical encounters. Over 70 specific diseases and environmental exposures are reported to each service's independent reportable event system, which captures these and additional service-specific medical events. For each of the reportable events, a clear case definition, laboratory criteria for diagnosis, and associated ICD-9 code are specified to standardize reporting across DoD. Information on specified diseases, exposures, and conditions is reported to AFHSC and incorporated into DMSS, with the aim of enabling timely and adequate response, identification of emerging or re-emerging diseases, and estimation of disease distribution, trends, and risk across the military population.

Mortality Surveillance

The Global Emerging Infections Surveillance and Response System (GEIS) and the Armed Forces Institute of Pathology (AFIP) established a Mortality Surveillance Division in the Office of the Armed Forces Medical Examiner. The division was created in 2001 to track mortality among all military personnel and monitor cause-specific mortality among service members in near real time. It does not collect specimens on a routine or systematic basis for the purposes of surveillance. This system tracks DoD personnel casualty data, integrated from the four services, in close to real time through the Defense Casualty Information Processing System. Additionally, the Armed Forces Medical Examiner's Tracking System provides data for epidemiologic analysis and real-time surveillance of casualty trends. The system also archives all military personnel death certificates and autopsy reports.

Disease and Non-Battle Injury (DNBI) Surveillance

Disease and non-battle injury (DNBI) surveillance is required by the Joint Chiefs of Staff and performed by the COCOMs to document non-combat-related health events occurring in a theater of operations. Outpatient data are collected by Field Medics/Battalion Aid Stations (i.e., Level I), Division Level Health Support (i.e., Level II), and Corps Level Health Support (i.e., Level III). Inpatient data are collected by Levels II–III. Data are collected through patient encounter modules and fed into JMeWS. Patient encounter modules (e.g., within the Armed Forces Health Longitudinal Technology Application—Theater system), are used to capture data such as individually identifying information (name, Social Security number, unit, etc.) and ICD-9 diagnostic codes. Data are generally aggregated for reporting purposes. Although there are instances where it is not feasible (e.g., where classified data transmission lines are not available, or in systems that cannot capture patient encounters), generally JMeWS is considered the primary source for data reporting. Because JMeWS is a classified information system, it is precluded from direct connection and data sharing with the DMSS, which is currently an unclassified system. The COCOM surgeons monitor DNBI trends and report threats to the Joint Staff and the services and components (JCS, 2007, Enclosure C). At least through early 2008, personnel at the ASD(HA) reviewed DNBI data on a daily basis; we understand that this function has been incorporated into the new AFHSC since February 2008, when this study concluded.[1]

Individual Medical Readiness (IMR)

DoD policy assigns responsibility and establishes procedures to improve individual medical readiness (IMR) through monitoring and reporting of a common set of indicators for all services (DoDI 6025.19 and DoDD 5124.2). The medical readiness of active component service members and select reserve component military personnel is assessed continuously and provides the basis for ensuring a force that is medically ready to deploy.

The six elements identified for monitoring medical readiness for deployment, and the standard for each, are: (1) a periodic health assessment (annual), (2) the absence of deployment-limiting conditions, (3) dental readiness (class 1 or 2 per annual dental exam[2]), (4) immunization status (current for total force/all services vaccines), (5) medical readiness laboratory tests (HIV test results on file within past 24 months, and a one-time DNA specimen), and (6) individual medical equipment (nuclear, biological, and chemical protective mask inserts for deployable members needing visual correction) (DoDI 6025.19, para 6.1). Services may enhance these basic requirements, although they are not required to report any of the data derived from enhanced monitoring.

The services report their data to the ASD(HA), which oversees the entire program and has the responsibility to issue periodic medical readiness reports (DoDI 6025.19, para 5.1.4). Services currently report IMR via the Status of Resources and Training System, though it is expected to migrate to the new readiness reporting system called

---

[1]   Personal communication to authors, October 15, 2007, and July 28, 2008.

[2]   The classes of dental readiness are as follows: class 1 = exam is current, no follow-up needed; class 2 = exam is current, only minor follow-up needed but it is not expected to be urgent in the next 12 months; class 3 = exam is current, urgent or emergent treatment needed; class 4 = exam is overdue or not current.

the Defense Readiness Reporting System, once available. Individual service commanders have full visibility and access to respective force medical readiness data through service-specific IMR program applications.

Key Organizational Components and Programs

To understand the current and potential utility of DoDSR and DMSS to surveillance, investigation, and research activities, the RAND team gathered information about ongoing surveillance by DoD organizations that play key roles in military public health activities. We interviewed military public health leaders and reviewed official documents and scientific publications to complement interview data.

The following sections provide brief overviews of the organizations, their respective roles in DoD medical surveillance, activities related to influenza specifically, and collaborations with or use of the DoDSR and/or DMSS. Figure 3.1, which was derived from multiple DoD web pages, depicts these organizational components within the overall DoD organizational structure, prior to establishment of the new AFHSC.

Global Emerging Infections Surveillance and Response System (GEIS)

The Global Emerging Infections Surveillance and Response System (GEIS) was created as a tri-service organizational entity located within the U.S. Army. As of February 2008, GEIS now falls under the purview of the new AFHSC. The origins of GEIS trace back to a September 1995 interagency report on global emerging infectious diseases (National Science and Technology Council, 1995) and an August 1995 memorandum from the Commanding General of the Army Medical Research and Materiel Command.[3] On October 10, 1995, the ASD(HA) announced the assembly of a Global Surveillance and Response Committee to develop a charter and provide oversight for a DoD global surveillance and response capability. The system was subsequently formalized by Presidential Decision Directive NSTC-7 (Emerging Infectious Diseases) in 1996 (PDD, 1996), which expanded the role of DoD in worldwide surveillance and response to emerging infectious diseases.

Citing the HIV/AIDS pandemic and the re-emergence of tuberculosis, cholera and pneumonia, the directive stipulated that "the mission of DoD will be expanded to include support of global surveillance, training research, and response to emerging infectious disease threats" (para 8). It further specified that DoD centrally coordinate

---

[3]   The memorandum included the following:

In response to the Office of Science and Technology Policy within the Executive Office of the President and to a request by the Office of the Assistant Secretary of Defense (Health Affairs), the U.S. Army Medical Research and Material Command and the Naval Medical Research and Development Command are initiating a program on global surveillance for emerging infectious diseases. This initiative relies heavily on the overseas laboratories.

Personal communication with Dr. Patrick Kelley, April 22, 2008.

Figure 3.1
Organizational Context for Military Health Surveillance

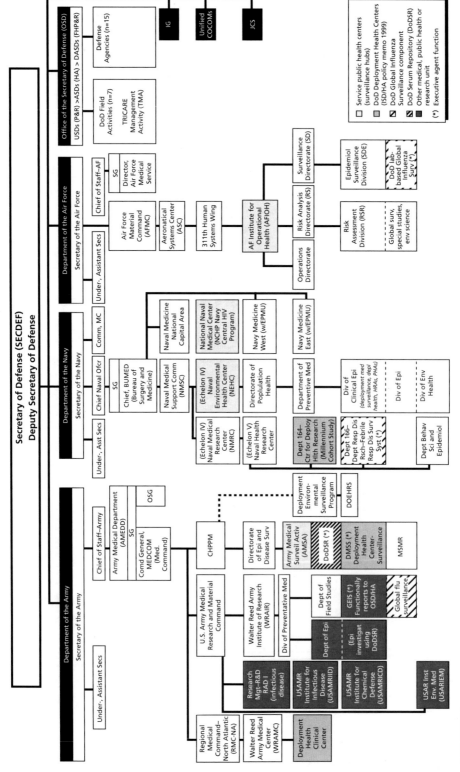

RAND MG875-3.1

the effort, improve its preventive health and epidemiologic capacities, and increase the use of existing CONUS and OCONUS facilities. Further, DoD was directed to use its overseas facilities to train foreign epidemiological staff. The goals of GEIS include surveillance and detection, response and readiness, integration and innovation, and cooperation and capacity building.

GEIS supports health surveillance programs and activities focusing on the following conditions: respiratory illnesses (including influenza), other febrile illnesses (malaria and dengue), enteric illnesses (acute diarrhea), antimicrobial resistance, and sexually transmitted infections. The GEIS-sponsored Mortality Surveillance Division is run by the AFIP Medical Examiner's Office and collects tri-service casualty information in near real time. The ESSENCE syndromic surveillance system, an outbreak detection tool monitoring daily garrison-based outpatient medical encounters, also receives support from GEIS.

Influenza surveillance programs sponsored by GEIS are primarily laboratory based. They focus on collection and characterization of viral isolates sampled from military and civilian populations from approximately 273 participating sites in 56 countries in FY06, with an additional 38 sites in nine countries that were added in FY07. Permanent overseas medical research laboratories are located in Egypt, Indonesia, Kenya, Peru, and Thailand and serve as collaborative centers with host nation research entities, the World Health Organization, and the Centers for Disease Control and Prevention. These research centers host the GEIS surveillance functions for DoD.

GEIS and DoDSR, DMSS. GEIS's collaborative efforts with AMSA (before the creation of the AFHSC) and the DoDSR and DMSS resources under AMSA management focused on supporting research and "threat assessments" or investigations. A number of studies involving military and civilian researchers have been sponsored by GEIS (DoD–GEIS Annual Report, 2006). For example, a recent suspected outbreak of Q-Fever among Army service members stationed in Iraq was investigated drawing on historical serum specimens from the DoDSR. In addition to collaborative work, GEIS used avian/pandemic influenza funding in late 2007 to provide infrastructure support to the DoDSR, through the purchase of a specimen transport truck for the use of a contractor to enable more timely shipment of serum specimens from contract testing facilities to the DoDSR.

Center for Health Promotion and Preventive Medicine (CHPPM)

The U.S. Army Center for Health Promotion and Preventive Medicine (CHPPM) acts as the Army's public health center and is the designated executive agent for health surveillance (DoDD 6490.2). Its mission is "to provide worldwide technical support for implementing preventive medicine, public health, and health promotion/wellness services in all aspects of America's Army and the Army Community anticipating and rapidly responding to operational needs and adaptable to a changing world environment." Designated CHPPM in 1994, the organization provides scientific expertise and services in clinical and field preventive medicine, environmental and occupational health, health promotion and wellness, epidemiology and disease surveillance, toxicology, and related laboratory sciences.

Prior to the creation of the new AFHSC in early 2008, CHPPM was organized into eight directorates, with the Directorate of Epidemiology and Disease Surveillance (DEDS) providing the central epidemiologic resource for the Army; AMSA was one of five programs within DEDS. Other directorates specialize in environmental health engineering, health promotion and wellness, health risk management, laboratory sciences, occupational and environmental medicine, occupational health sciences, and toxicology.

As described in other sections, management and oversight of DoDSR and DMSS had been the responsibility of AMSA and now fall under the new AFHSC.

CHPPM and DoDSR, DMSS. According to AMSA analysts, there have been limited formal mechanisms for making data within DMSS available for use by CHPPM personnel outside of AMSA. Further, CHPPM and its component directorates do not regularly utilize the contents of the DoDSR for surveillance purposes. Given DMSS and the DoDSR's current physical set-up and geographic remoteness to most of CHPPM staff and facilities, use of these resources requires onsite staff in order to access data and specimens.

Air Force Institute for Operational Health (AFIOH)

The Air Force Institute for Operational Health (AFIOH) acts as the public health center for the U.S. Air Force and provides occupational, environmental, and public health expertise to operational decisionmakers and policymakers. AFIOH is the executive agent for the laboratory-based component of the virologic surveillance activities supported by GEIS and is under the command of the 311th Human Services Wing.

The AFIOH consists of five divisions, of which two are directly engaged in surveillance: the Risk Analysis Directorate and the Surveillance Directorate. The Risk Analysis Directorate collects and analyzes environmental, safety, and health data in order to enhance performance and protect the force. The Surveillance Directorate collects data on personnel health such as HIV status and drug testing for the Air Force. It also provides chemistry services for air, soil, and water analysis as well as expertise and analytic services for surveillance of radiation.

The AFIOH laboratory-based surveillance program collects specimens from participating care facilities and sentinel sites around the world. A total of 43 U.S. Military Treatment Facilities (MTFs) located worldwide collect specimens from DoD beneficiaries attending hospitals, health clinics, emergency clinics, and pediatric clinics; other sentinel sites include two military hospitals in Hungary serving foreign military beneficiaries and multiple treatment facilities in 13 allied countries serving foreign military and civilian patients. Overseas GEIS laboratories also work closely in support of the AFIOH lab-based surveillance program, through specimen collection and testing.

AFIOH and DoDSR, DMSS. Currently, the AFIOH sends remnant serum from HIV screening, HIV test results, and reportable medical events captured in garrison to DoDSR and DMSS.

Navy Environmental Health Center (NEHC)

The Navy Environmental Health Center (NEHC) serves as the public health center for the U.S. Navy and Marine Corps and is under the Navy Medical Support Command. NEHC's mission is to "provide leadership and expertise to ensure mission readiness through disease prevention and health promotion in support of the National Military Strategy" (NEHC, 2008). NEHC is made up of the five following directorates: Environmental Programs, Expeditionary Preventive Medicine, Industrial Hygiene, Occupational and Environmental Medicine, and Population Health. Thus, NEHC addresses the full range of health surveillance components, including medical surveillance and occupational and environmental surveillance.

NEHC's EpiData Center provides epidemiologic services in support of the Navy's disease and injury prevention programs. It conducts infectious disease and deployment health surveillance, and it provides clinical epidemiology, occupational and environmental epidemiology, and injury epidemiology analytic services.

Currently the EpiData Center receives HL-7 data feeds of pathogen laboratory results from medical specimens, blood chemistry results, and pharmacy data and has the capability of linking these data streams to health outcomes within the electronic medical record system. The center plans to test the integration potential of these HL-7 data sources to the ESSENCE syndromic surveillance system to provide validation of diagnoses coded by outpatient ICD-9 codes.

NEHC and the DoDSR, DMSS. Currently, NEHC sends remnant sera from HIV screening, deployment-related health assessment forms DD 2795, DD 2796, and DD 2900, and reportable medical events captured in garrison to DoDSR and DMSS, respectively. As of January 2008, when this study concluded, AMSA reportedly had not received HIV positivity/negativity data related to the specimens in its current inventory from the Navy ViroMed contract. Further, NEHC provides data to the DMSS, though it has had little need for DMSS analysis or specimens to date.

Naval Health Research Center (NHRC)

The Naval Health Research Center is the research hub for the U.S. Navy and Marine Corps. NHRC is made up of the following six departments: Medical Modeling, Simulation and Mission Support, Warfighter Performance, Behavioral Sciences and Epidemiology, Deployment Health Research, HIV/AIDS Programs, and Respiratory Diseases Research. NHRC serves as one of three designated deployment health centers: the Center for Deployment Health Research (ASD(HA), September 30, 1999).

NHRC serves as the Navy node for GEIS and conducts active surveillance of febrile respiratory illness (FRI) in recruit training centers DoD-wide, on board ships, and in local border areas (San Diego–Mexican border). Additionally, as part of the FRI surveillance program, NHRC collects and tests throat swabs for adenovirus and influenza virus, employing molecular techniques for pathogen isolation, characterization, and preservation. NHRC archives throat swab specimens and isolates from this surveillance program in frozen storage at –80°C.

The Naval Respiratory Disease Laboratory, part of the DoD Center for Deployment Health Research at NHRC, has culture and molecular testing capabilities for approximately 21 bacterial, viral, and other respiratory pathogens including *Streptococcus pneumoniae, Streptococcus pyogenes,* influenza, adenovirus, and coronavirus. This laboratory also conducts serologic testing and is currently running serology for adenovirus, chlamydia, and *M. pneumoniae.*

NHRC and DoDSR, DMSS. NHRC collaborated closely with AMSA on ad hoc research studies and has utilized DoDSR serum and DMSS data for studies of special interest (e.g., acute respiratory infections among military recruits). No formal standing mechanism existed between NHRC and AMSA for purposes of exchanging data or conducting surveillance; RAND is unaware of any changes in status since the creation of the AFHSC after this study was completed.

Chapter Highlights

- Medical surveillance within the DoD is accomplished at many levels, across all services, and through numerous different systems. Not surprisingly, data systems are stovepiped within services and segregated by garrison or theater context, with data classification compounding connectivity issues.
- There is strong evidence that medical surveillance within DoD is hampered by lack of data sharing, lack of timely data, and even missing data, such as the location of individuals in a theater of operations. In spite of the fact that Congress has directed DoD to solve the location data problem, the DMSS is not yet receiving any feeds at the individual level because the one service-specific system with this information is classified and DMSS is not.
- Further, there appears to be a difference between policy and practice in terms of which DoD surveillance system and organization should be tracking this information.

CHAPTER FOUR

Current Capabilities of AMSA, DoDSR, and DMSS

In this chapter we highlight the operations and capabilities of AMSA, the DoDSR, and DMSS up until the creation of the AFHSC in late February 2008. For DMSS in particular, we examine capabilities against the requirements described in Chapter Two. Together with the examination of other biological specimen repositories, which is the focus of Chapter Five, this information establishes the basis for the analysis of issues, gaps, and opportunities to improve the capabilities of AMSA, DoDSR, and DMSS, which is the focus of Chapter Six.

The Army Medical Surveillance Activity

AMSA, a component of CHPPM (see Figure 4.1), has been the DoD's source for medical surveillance information and analysis. AMSA's budget was approximately $4 million per year, according to our interview sources, and covered the cost of AMSA staff, the DoDSR, and DMSS management and operations. AMSA's mission statement was as follows:

> The Army Medical Surveillance Activity's (AMSA) main functions are to analyze, interpret, and disseminate information regarding the status, trends, and determinants of the health and fitness of U.S. military (and military-associated) populations and to identify and evaluate obstacles to medical readiness. AMSA is the central epidemiological resource for the U.S. Armed Forces providing regularly scheduled and customer-requested analyses and reports to policy makers, medical planners, and researchers. It identifies and evaluates obstacles to medical readiness by linking various databases that communicate information relevant to service members' experience that has the potential to affect their health. (AMSA Mission, personal correspondence, January 28, 2008)

AMSA's mission statement did not capture explicitly all core functions. Although the executive agency for AMSA clearly describes the organization's mission in terms of deployment medical surveillance, these assigned requirements did not appear in AMSA's own mission statement. In fact, AMSA's mission seemed focused on medical

Figure 4.1
Chain of Command for AMSA

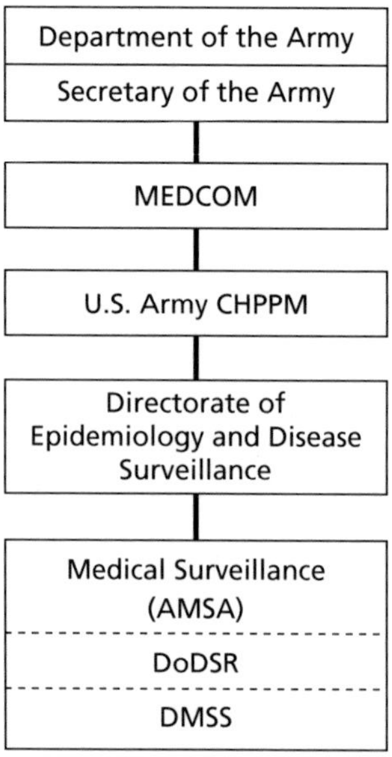

```
┌─────────────────────────────────┐
│     Department of the Army      │
│     Secretary of the Army       │
└─────────────────────────────────┘
             │
┌─────────────────────────────────┐
│            MEDCOM               │
└─────────────────────────────────┘
             │
┌─────────────────────────────────┐
│        U.S. Army CHPPM          │
└─────────────────────────────────┘
             │
┌─────────────────────────────────┐
│        Directorate of           │
│   Epidemiology and Disease      │
│         Surveillance            │
└─────────────────────────────────┘
             │
┌─────────────────────────────────┐
│      Medical Surveillance       │
│            (AMSA)               │
│- - - - - - - - - - - - - - - - -│
│            DoDSR                │
│- - - - - - - - - - - - - - - - -│
│            DMSS                 │
└─────────────────────────────────┘
```

RAND *MG875-4.1*

NOTE: This was the organizational structure before the creation of the AFHSC in late February 2008, after this study was completed.

readiness and the "health and fitness" of military populations. The word "surveillance," what staff described as AMSA's core function, does not appear in the mission statement.

AMSA staff included assigned military officers, civilian General Service staff, and contractor personnel working for the five principal contracts. Among military officers, there were positions for a Chief (Army O5-6 Preventive Medicine Physician), Preventive Medicine Officers (two Army O3-4 Preventive Medicine Physicians), and Service Liaison Officers (currently one Air Force O5 Preventive Medicine Physician, with one Navy position unfilled).

As we have already established, AMSA had responsibility to manage both the DoDSR and the DMSS, and the new AFHSC has now incorporated this responsibility. AFHSC now also manages a data tool called the Defense Medical Epidemiology Database (DMED) that provides remote access to a subset of DMSS data. AMSA supported a number of contracts to help manage the repository, DMSS, and analyses:

- DMED contract: responsible for maintaining internal applications (the DoDSR inventory management application, the DMSS management tool application) and external user applications, as well as facilitating provision of technical data extracts to external customers.

- DMSS contract: responsible for maintaining and developing DMSS, which includes acquisition and loading of data, software development, and maintenance of hardware.
- DoDSR contract: responsible for maintenance of the DoDSR freezers and supporting infrastructure (e.g., compressors, backup generators) and the daily operations of the DoDSR, which include the processing of new specimens and the retrieval of specimens and their aliquoting for external study. This contract is also responsible for specimen pickup from the sources, which requires a specialized transport truck.
- Two separate analysis contracts: support staff analysts for internally directed analyses and external research requests, including serum studies.

DoD Serum Repository

The DoDSR stores sera from service members' blood. The basic serum storage process stems from the original purpose of the repository, which was to collect and store sera collected as a result of HIV testing. AMSA ran the serum repository via contracts, which involved specimen collection, transport, and storage. AMSA made serum available to military and civilian researchers for "purposes of conducting military relevant investigations" and regulated the use according to official AMSA guidelines (AMSA, 2003). We are unaware of any changes that may have been made in these procedures by the new AFHSC, since this organization was created after completion of our study.

The repository contains specimens received from two main sources: the department-wide HIV screening programs (DoDD 6485.1) and deployment-related health assessments (DoDI 6490.03). The repository has received remnant serum from the HIV testing programs of the Army, Navy, and Military Entrance Processing Stations since 1985 and serum specimens from the Air Force HIV testing program since 1996.

On average, the repository grows by an additional 1.9 million specimens per year and includes specimens collected from service members stationed domestically and in Europe. As of December 2007, the repository included a total inventory of over 43 million serum specimens collected from approximately 10.5 million individuals (see Table 4.1). Of these, an estimated 2,628 were known to be HIV positive specimens. However, most positive specimens are retained by the services or by the Army's retrovirology laboratory at WRAIR.

Of the 43.1 million specimens, approximately 37.6 million are linked to personnel data and are available for immediate physical retrieval from frozen storage. Of those, approximately 13.7 million specimens are from the 2.2 million individuals currently in the service (as of October 31, 2007).

Table 4.1
Description of DoDSR Serum Inventory and Source of Specimens

DoDSR contents	
Total number of specimens*	43,194,251
Total number of individuals	10,418,551
Acquisition rate	1.9 million per year
Source of specimens	
Current active duty**	1,402,589
Current reservist members	375,012
Current National Guard	456,183
Former military members	5,001,228
Dependant beneficiaries	898,358
Median number of specimens per service member	
Current active duty	6 (IQR 3,9)
Current reservists	6 (IQR 3,9)
Current National Guard members	5 (IQR 2,7)
Number of known HIV+ specimens	2,628

* As of December 31, 2007.
** As of October 31, 2007.
IQR = interquartile range.

As a result of storage space restrictions at the current DoDSR facilities, approximately 5.5 million specimens for which no linked data currently exist (i.e., the specimen is not linked to an individual SSN) have been placed in "compressed configuration." Much of the information needed to link these specimens to individual SSNs exists currently on paper manifests, which are awaiting either verification of manual transcription or initial manual transcription. Entry of these data is awaiting contract award. Of the approximately 5.5 million specimens in "compressed configuration," only 244,876 are from the 2.2 million individuals currently in the service (as of October 31, 2007).

Also as of 2007, serum specimens are shipped to the DoDSR from three laboratories: ViroMed Laboratories (Minnetonka, Minnesota), with which the Army and Navy each has a contract, and the Air Force Institute for Operational Health (San Antonio, Texas). Specimens from COCOMs, such as those coming from the Landstuhl Regional Medical Center (Ramstein, Germany), are shipped to the serum repository via the Walter Reed Army Institute of Research. Specimens from ViroMed and AFIOH have been transported routinely by a contract carrier to the DoDSR approximately six times per year.

Specimens are stored at –30°C in 25,000 square feet of leased walk-in freezers, which are now nearly full. The lease for this space expires in 2010, and we learned from our interviews that AMSA was in the process of defining its future storage requirements.

Source of Specimens

Seventy-five percent of service members have provided three or more specimens. Serial collection of serum specimens is an important feature of the repository because it permits longitudinal studies capable of assessing temporal trends as well as long-term health effects in individuals and population cohorts. Thus, the number of consecutive specimens contributed by a given service member determines to a great extent the epidemiologic utility of the stored specimens. As shown in Table 4.1, as of October 2007, the median number of specimens per active component and reserve component service member was 6 (IQR 3,9). Thus, approximately 75 percent of active component and reservist service members had provided three or more specimens. For the National Guard, the median number of specimens contributed was 5 (IQR 2,7).

Over half the specimens are traceable to service members who have been on active duty after 1990. According to AMSA analysts, over half of the serum specimens in the DoDSR are traceable to a service member who has at some point been on active duty after 1990. As previously discussed, this subset of the population captured by the DoDSR is of high value because of the availability of linked longitudinal medical and personnel information. The total number of former and current military members represented in the DoDSR, including the current active component and reserve component members (as of October 31, 2007) is 7.2 million, and is the largest subpopulation making up the full pool of contributors to the serum repository (see Figure 4.2).

Specimens for civilian military applicants are also stored in the DoDSR. In addition to military service members, beneficiaries and civilian military applicants also contribute serum specimens to the DoDSR. Civilians applying for military service are required to be tested for serologic evidence of HIV-1 infection (DoDD 6485.1) as a criterion for eligibility for service. These specimens are stored in the DoDSR because testing contracts include packaging and shipment of all specimens tested for HIV-1 irrespective of military duty status. Since 1998, reserve component members have had the same blood collection requirements as active component members, including routine HIV screening and pre- and post-deployment specimens (ASD(HA), October 6, 1998). Approximately 2.3 million individuals with specimens in the repository are classified as unidentifiable (see Figure 4.2). According to AMSA analysts, the majority of unidentifiable specimens are from civilian applicants who did not join the military and a small number of affiliated civilians who had received HIV testing pre- or post-deployment.

Consent forms are not needed when the sample is taken. Consent issues arise twice: first at the time of the taking of the blood specimen, and second when uses of stored sera are proposed. Blood is drawn from service members for both HIV testing and for pre- and post-deployment specimens, with the HIV test specimen serving as the deployment-related specimen when it meets certain criteria described in DoDI 6490.03. According to our interviews, there are no consent forms needed from service members at the time of taking these specimens, since the specimen collections are done

Figure 4.2
Contributors to the DoDSR (as of October 31, 2007)

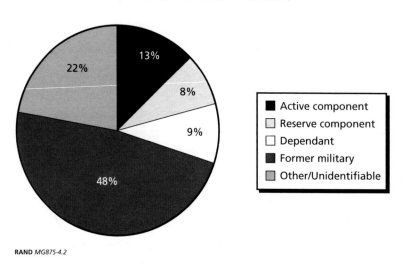

RAND *MG875-4.2*

for public health surveillance and as a condition of employment in the service. Second, serum specimens are stored in perpetuity in the DoDSR, with no apparent guidelines governing appropriate handling and/or disposal of sera from separated or deceased members. Our interviewees suggested that service members know that their serum specimens are stored in perpetuity; however, we could find no evidence of explicit communication to that effect.

Guidelines address uses of stored serum specimens, but consent rules are not fully articulated. For uses of the serum specimens, AMSA's "Guidelines for Collecting, Maintaining, Requesting, and Using Specimens Stored in the Department of Defense Serum Repository," (May 29, 2003) established "research" as an activity conducted with the primary intent to create, extend, or validate generalizable knowledge, or knowledge that extends beyond the individual (or populations directly associated with the individual). "Nonresearch" is an activity conducted in order to develop specific knowledge of an individual or directly associated population. Within these two categories, the guidelines addressed four primary uses of the stored serum specimens: research, patient care, public health/force health protection, and criminal investigations. The issue of consent was addressed by determining whether the sera are identifiable to an individual (i.e., linked) or unidentifiable:

- For research purposes, linked specimens would require consent documents, and unlinked specimens would not require consent.
- For patient care purposes, a consent must be obtained prior to specimen release.
- For public health/force health protection, linked specimens would not require consent if the use is "nonresearch" and if the use is to examine a threat to or inter-

vention for a military population. The guideline did not describe when linked specimens might require consent for the purposes of public health/force health protection. However, it did describe the potential use of an unlinked specimen, although it was not explicit about whether this use would or would not require consent (presumably it would not).

- For criminal investigations and prosecutions, the guidelines were quiet concerning the need for consent, although they specify the use of counsel.

It appears that the guidelines could be improved upon by specifying consent issues relating to public health/force health protection. Further, from the discussion above, since the specimens are drawn without consent, there seemed to be no way to use the sera for any purposes other than "delinked" or certain public health/force health protection uses.

Guidelines for use of institutional review boards (IRBs) could be expanded. We learned from our interviews that AMSA relies on the IRBs of requesting agencies to determine the appropriateness of the protections stipulated within the proposed protocols, although the current trend among repositories is to have an internal IRB or an established affiliation with an IRB (see Chapter Five). As in our discussion of informed consent above, because recent technological innovations allow for detection of DNA in sera, it is questionable whether sera can actually be "delinked." The AMSA guidelines specified the following IRB requirements for proposed uses of sera:

- For research purposes, AMSA required an IRB approval.
- For the purposes of patient care, the AMSA guideline was silent on the matter of IRB approval.
- For the purposes of public health/force health protection, the guidelines were silent with regard to IRB approval, although this category of use in particular may warrant an IRB.
- For the purposes of criminal investigations and prosecutions, the guidelines were also silent, although they stipulate the use of counsel.

Therefore, guidelines articulating the protections offered by an IRB review may be improved upon by further detailing when an IRB is going to be used, and which IRB will be used (i.e., either an AMSA/AFHSC-affiliated IRB or the requesting organization's IRB).

There appear to be several opportunities for improvement in the treatment and description of the requirements for an IRB as well as informed consent, and this suggests that an updated examination might provide benefit both to the service member as well as to the Military Health System.

To summarize the key points of this discussion regarding informed consent:

- Specimens are being drawn for two legally mandated and regulated purposes: HIV testing and pre- and post-deployment surveillance.
- Specimens are stored in perpetuity with no evidence of communication of that to service members.
- Specimens can be used for purposes other than that for which they were drawn (namely research, clinical care, public health, and criminal investigation), but research uses require either delinking from individually identifying information or express informed consent.
- The consent rules were apparently not fully articulated in AMSA guidelines.

And, for the use of IRBs:

- Repositories either tend to be affiliated with existing IRBs or they constitute their own internal IRBs. In contrast, AMSA relied exclusively on the determination of requesting organization IRBs.
- The guideline articulating the need for IRBs was silent in the case of using sera for public health/force health protection. Because this category of use is large, it may benefit AFHSC to revisit this use of serum specimens and further specify the appropriateness of if, when, and how to use an IRB.

Timing of Specimen Collection

The events associated with specimen collection and subsequent storage by the DoDSR include: application for military service, routine HIV screening, deployment-related health assessments (both before and after) and separation from military service. Individual medical readiness requirements (DoDI 6025.19) also include compulsory HIV screening for all active component and reserve component members, with screening intervals not to exceed 24 months. Pre-deployment specimens must be collected no more than one year before deployment and post-deployment specimens within 30 days of redeployment home. Notably, specimens collected as part of medical encounters, in garrison or in theater, are not stored or sent to the DoDSR. Furthermore, blood collected as part of medical care provided by the Veterans Health Administration system is not currently required to be stored by the DoDSR.

Specimens

Specimens are kept in frozen storage. All domestically collected blood specimens are drawn at Military Treatment Facilities (MTFs), where they are spun down for serum extraction. The serum is packaged and shipped from MTFs to either ViroMed or AFIOH at a temperature of 4–8°C (usually 24–48 hours after the blood draw). At the testing laboratories, specimens are processed and tested for evidence of HIV antibody, using ELISA-based identification methods. Specimens are maintained at 4–8°C during the preparation and testing process. After testing, specimens are placed in frozen storage at –30°C at ViroMed and AFIOH testing facilities. From testing laboratories, remnant serum specimens from HIV screening are transferred by truck at –30°C to DoDSR six times per year.

Specimens collected from service members stationed overseas in Europe and Iraq are sent to Landstuhl Regional Medical Center, Germany. At Landstuhl, specimens are processed to serum, if not already done, and then frozen and shipped in batches to the HIV Diagnostic Reference Laboratory in the Division of Retrovirology at the Walter Reed Army Institute of Research. There, specimens are processed and tested for HIV infection. After testing, specimens are frozen and delivered on dry ice to the DoDSR on a weekly basis. Upon arrival at the DoDSR, they are scanned to verify arrival and entered into the DoDSR inventory program.

The HIV Diagnostic Reference Laboratory also acts as the quality assurance laboratory for the ViroMed contract. Management personnel in the HIV Diagnostic Reference Laboratory review digital images of all of the HIV positive specimens from ViroMed. If they do not concur on the diagnosis, verification testing is requested. The HIV Diagnostic Reference Laboratory also reviews any incident reports generated by ViroMed describing conditions or incidents occurring during the shipping and testing processes with the potential to influence diagnostic test results.

Currently, the HIV Diagnostic Reference Laboratory has no way to verify the cold chain for the serum specimens drawn in either the United States or Germany. Once a specimen is drawn, no standing mechanism exists to verify appropriate handling along the specimen's trajectory toward the ViroMed testing laboratory. The HIV testing protocol that is followed requires that specimens be tested within 2 to 7 days of being drawn, if the specimens are not frozen.

Uses of the Serum Repository

As of early February 2008, DoDSR had distributed specimens for over 170 different studies and clinical support needs. For nonmilitary related researchers to receive specimens, they must collaborate with a military principal investigator and go through the military IRB process. Costs associated with specimen use by nonmilitary researchers are $20 per specimen. Uses of the specimens for military-related research are exempt from the $20 fee. Approved research studies can receive only unidentified serum specimens. Use of unidentified serum specimens for research purposes precludes the linking of specimens to other individual-level demographic, medical, and personnel data stored in the DMSS database.[1]

---

[1] Research activities involving human subjects that are exempt from IRB review and the requirement for informed consent are identified in 45CFR 46.101(b)(1)–(6). In particular, 45CFR 46.101(b)(4) is relevant to the use of stored human specimens. It states:

> Research involving the collection or study of existing data, documents, records, pathological specimens, or diagnostic specimens, if these sources are publicly available or if the information is recorded by the investigator in such a manner that subjects cannot be identified, directly or through identifiers linked to the subjects.

AMSA did not publish a description of its decisionmaking process for approving use of the sera. According to this AMSA guideline, authority over the release of specimens and compliance with stated requirements was determined solely by the Director of AMSA. To our knowledge, AMSA did not publish the criteria or process it used in approving release of serum specimens. As specified in AMSA's "Guidelines for Collecting, Maintaining, Requesting and Using Specimens Stored in the Department of Defense Serum Repository" (AMSA, 2003), access to specimens was based on consideration of the following factors: nature of intended use, DoD affiliation, and number/size of specimens. Categories of intended use include: "research," "patient care," "public health/force health protection: community and military preventive care," and "criminal investigations and prosecutions." There was no separate category for "deployment health." Specific logistical and technical requirements were described in detail according to the category of intended use of the specimens.

To date, most uses of DoDSR have been for research rather than surveillance. According to DoD policy (ASD(HA), 2005 and DoDD 6490.2), serum collection and storage is intended to contribute to deployment-related surveillance, although the ability of serum to provide information on agents or exposure markers has yet to be explicitly defined or systematically evaluated. Further, there appears to be no ongoing body that systematically evaluates potential new exposure threats and improvements in technology to detect those threats in biological specimens against available resources.

Specimens stored at the DoDSR together with the service members' linked health and personnel information supply a robust resource for supporting surveillance, investigating outbreaks (especially for providing pre-exposure serum specimens for comparison with outbreak-associated specimens), addressing research questions, and supporting clinical management. Table 4.2 shows the number of distinct requests for serum specimens by year, and Table 4.3 shows the number of requests by type of use.

From January 2001 to January 2008, AMSA received only 122 requests for specimens from the DoDSR. The various uses of serum specimens are described in more detail in the following sections.

Surveillance. The only routine surveillance use of DoDSR remains the HIV screening program, despite what is called for by department policy regarding deployment health and the DoDSR's role. No other tests or analyses are routinely or systematically carried out on DoDSR specimens. According to AMSA analysts, AMSA was not resourced or funded to support regular or systematic analysis of pre- and post-deployment serum specimens (paired or otherwise) for the purpose of performing biological surveillance of deployment-related health threats. AMSA supported many

---

Therefore, as long as certain identifiers have been removed (i.e., the 18 identifiers specified under the Health Insurance Portability and Accountability Act at section 164.514(b)(2) of the regulations—i.e., name, Social Security number, medical record number, telephone number, email address, health plan beneficiary number, etc.), the specimen and any accompanying data can be considered de-identified and may be exempt from needing IRB oversight and informed consent.

**Table 4.2
Number of DoDSR Specimen Requests
(Military and Civilian), 2001 Through 2008**

Year	Number of Approved Serum Requests
2001	11
2002	17
2003	6
2004	11
2005	12
2006	19
2007	43
2008	3
Total	122

**Table 4.3
Uses of the Serum Inventory, 2001 Through February 2008**

Uses of Serum	Number of Approved Serum Requests
Vaccine	27
Clinical support	19
Deployment related	12
Miscellaneous	9
HIV	8
Epidemiologic investigation	7
Influenza	3
Seroprevalence	3
Forensic	2
Research (n = 32)	
Noncommunicable disease	18
Infectious disease	4
Miscellaneous	3
DNA	3
HIV	2
Drug	1
Chemical	1
Total	122

external requests for relatively small numbers of such paired specimens, focusing on specific time periods and locations and testing for specific exposures of interest, but this process did not result in a robust or systematic infrastructure for such biological surveillance. AMSA did not have its own laboratory capability to support such testing. This may trace back to the origins of the DoDSR as a repository for specimens already tested for HIV, rather than as a surveillance laboratory.

Investigation. AMSA was not resourced to conduct independent detection or response investigations to disease or injury outbreaks. AMSA's role in epidemiologic investigations was historically one of providing data and/or specimens in support of such investigations. A recent example is a Q-Fever outbreak among U.S. military troops returning from Iraq, in which AMSA was able to provide historical serum specimens as well as demographic and personnel information to assist in the investigation of the outbreak. Other examples include epidemiological investigation of outbreaks caused by influenza and adenovirus.

Research. To date, military public health and medical research account for the largest number of requests for specimens from DoDSR. Research projects for which specimens have been requested span a wide range of medical topics, including infectious diseases, cancers, diabetes, multiple sclerosis, and schizophrenia. Civilian and military researchers in the fields of immunology, infectious disease, cancer, cardiovascular epidemiology, nutrition, environmental health, and maternal/child health have tapped into this unique biological resource, as evidenced by the list of published reports found in Appendix B to this report, a bibliography of peer-reviewed scientific publications utilizing the DoDSR serum specimens or DMSS database. As discussed in prior sections, use of the serum for research purposes was stated in AMSA guidelines and needed to meet specific requirements for approved use. From 2001 through early February 2008, AMSA received approximately 120 requests for serum specimens, including approximately 30 research projects. Two research projects focused specifically on avian and/or pandemic influenza.

Clinical Support. Less taxing requests on specimens are made by clinicians to validate HIV test results or to obtain patient medical history information. Specimens requested to meet this need typically require less time and effort to process.

Avian and Pandemic Influenza. A particular focus of this study was use of the repository to address issues related to influenza.[2] Routine uses of the DoDSR and DMSS specific to influenza have not been established; however, beginning in FY06, three serologic studies investigated the utility of the DoDSR's serum inventory for surveillance of avian and pandemic influenza. We describe these in further detail below.

Seroprevalence of H5N1 antibody among service members deployed to countries with human H5N1 infections. Utilizing pre- and post- deployment health assessment forms and deployment rosters, AMSA was able to identify a cohort of 1,000 service members who deployed to Thailand, Indonesia, Vietnam, or Cambodia during periods when there were avian and human H5N1 cases among the local population. AMSA linked the deployment data to specimens in the repository for which the pre-

---

[2] The study was supported by pandemic influenza preparedness funds.

deployment specimen was drawn prior to the deployment and the post-deployment specimen was drawn within 365 days of return. Specimens were sent to the Southern Research Institute, where hemagglutination inhibition assays and confirmatory micro-neutralization assays for H5N1 Clade 1 and 2 viruses were performed. Results showed that approximately 1 percent of the study population was seropositive to H5 antibody prior to deployment, likely due to cross-reactive antibody. Out of the 1,000 subjects tested, only 2 subjects seroconverted during deployment to Thailand using a 1:40 antibody titer cutoff. No known exposures or respiratory illnesses were reported for these two subjects during or after the deployment. These cases of seroconversion may be due to cross-reactive antibody or false positives. Overall, AMSA investigators found no significant risk of H5N1 infection during deployments to countries with human H5N1 activity.

Evidence of prior immunity against influenza among recruits. A random sample was identified with 1,000 recruits who had a MEPS specimen collected in 2005. Serum specimens were tested for evidence of previous infection by the influenza H3 and H1 strains circulating during the previous year. The Southern Research Institute tested the specimens by hemagglutination inhibition assay. Results showed that approximately 43 percent and 66 percent of recruits were seropositive for H1 and H3 antibody, respectively. Thirty-two percent of recruits were seropositive for antibody to both viruses. No seasonality for seropositivity to either virus was found. Assessment of demographic and geographic factors associated with seropositivity was reported ongoing through February 2008.

Prolonged cough in service members deployed to Afghanistan. In early 2007, anecdotal reports from U.S. health care providers in Afghanistan surfaced that a large number of U.S. service members were experiencing prolonged episodes of cough. These reports led to the consideration of widespread administration of the new acellular pertussis vaccine. In response, preventive medicine assets at U.S. Central Command (CENTCOM) and Afghanistan asked AMSA and GEIS to conduct serological testing to determine the likely etiology prior to determination of vaccine policy. A study was initiated using pre- and post-deployment serum specimens to determine the seroconversion due to common respiratory pathogens during deployment to Afghanistan. Specifically, the seroprevalence of IgG and IgA antibody to *Chlamydia pneumoniae, Mycoplasma pneumoniae, Bordetella pertussis,* and parainfluenza virus (PIV), the seroprevalence of IgG and IgM antibody to adenovirus and respiratory syncytial virus (RSV), and the seroprevalence of hemagglutination inhibition antibody to influenza among U.S. military service members before and after deployment are being determined.

The results will serve to inform military vaccination and force health protection policy and should serve as a basis to set priorities among DoD respiratory pathogen research in the future.

Military and civilian researchers are the main users of the DoDSR. In addition to AMSA analysts and service public health surveillance hubs, military and civilian researchers make up the main user group of DoDSR specimens. Within the DoD, researchers and policymakers from the following organizations have used specimens from the serum collection: Walter Reed Army Institute of Research, the U.S. Army Medical Research Institute for Infectious Diseases, the Military Vaccine Agency, the Global Emerging Infections Surveillance and Response System, the Air Force Institute for Operational Health, the Navy Environmental Health Center, and the Naval Health Research Center. Because remote access to DMSS is not authorized, nor is it technically efficient with existing architecture, requests for data or specimens submitted by both internal (i.e., AMSA/AFHSC) and external (i.e., unaffiliated) entities and specimens are subject to the same review and handling process.

Defense Medical Surveillance System

As described earlier, in 1997 DMSS was created out of the existing Army Medical Surveillance System to provide tri-service medical surveillance. DMSS is a relational database that links individual health, personnel, and serologic data together to support department-wide public health and preventive medicine operations, and which is to receive "[a]ll theater medical surveillance and treatment data collected by the services, the Unified and Specified Commands, and the individual commands with the Services" (ASD(HA), September 30 1999, para 5).

The DMSS is a longitudinal surveillance database. As such, it is a unique tool because it relates service member–level information from various DoD sources and retains a longitudinal record spanning an individual's service career. The Defense Medical Epidemiology Database (DMED) is derived from DMSS, providing select DMSS data that are de-identified and remotely accessible to DoD members outside of AMSA/AFHSC. Figure 4.3 depicts the chronology over which the various data elements became integrated into the DMSS

DMSS has gradually integrated a broader range of data. The Army Medical Surveillance System, the predecessor of DMSS, was brought online in 1990; it became the DMSS in 1997. Since 1990, the database has gradually integrated a broader range of data from individual service members into a permanent central longitudinal data store and to date includes 401 million rows of information, including:

- Results from HIV tests.
- Information on applicants and inductees to military service from Military Entrance Processing Stations (MEPS).
- Immunizations.

- Casualty information. (According to AMSA analysts, transmission of casualty data to DMSS was discontinued in 2003 because of security concerns related to Operation Iraqi Freedom.)
- Personnel and demographic data (all persons in the active and reserve components, and civilian applicants).
- Inpatient medical encounter data for the active component.
- Deployment rosters for the first Gulf War and major deployments since then.
- Health assessment questionnaires administered before and after major deployments (DD Forms 2795, 2796, and 2900).
- Reportable medical events (in garrison).
- Outpatient medical encounter data for the active component.
- Characteristics of the serum repository specimens.

As of January 2008, 311 million rows of data in the aforementioned categories have been validated as belonging to identified military service members (the remaining data are from separated service members, beneficiaries, and nonmilitary member applicants).

HIV test results from contract testing laboratories are fed into DMSS weekly and the data reach back to 1985. DMSS receives its information on military applicants and inductees from the Military Entrance Processing Command for all services on a monthly basis and has data archived starting in 1985 (and continuing to the present). The Defense Enrollment Eligibility Reporting System has provided immunization data to DMSS for all services on a monthly basis since 1990, and data were retrospectively loaded, reaching back to 1980. The Defense Manpower Data Center provides monthly

Figure 4.3
Data Integrated into DMSS from Inception to December 2007

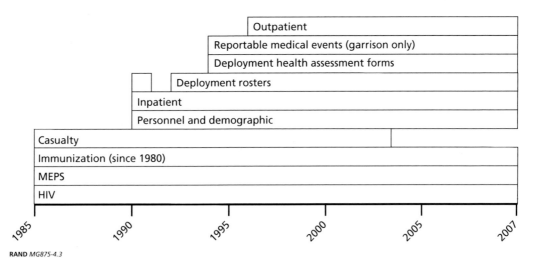

feeds to DMSS of personnel and demographic information and deployment roster files for all services from 1990 to 2007. DoD's Executive Information Decision Support sends inpatient and outpatient data files to DMSS on a daily basis for all services and has these data archived from 1990 and 1996, respectively, with outpatient data arriving on a monthly basis for outsourced care. Health assessment forms completed pre- and post-deployment have been included in DMSS since 1994 for all services. MTFs have provided reportable medical events data captured in garrison to DMSS daily since 1994.

MTFs have provided reportable medical events data captured in garrison to DMSS daily since 1994. HIV test results from contract testing laboratories are fed into DMSS weekly and the data reach back to 1985.

The Defense Enrollment Eligibility Reporting System has provided immunization data to DMSS for all services on a monthly basis since 1990, and data were retrospectively loaded, reaching back to 1980.

Comparison of Surveillance Data Requirements and DMSS Capabilities

A review of DoD policy (DoDD 6490.2 and DoDI 6490.03) reveals only very limited detail on the exact data elements required to fulfill all medical surveillance requirements. To review quickly, the mission of the DMSS was articulated in 1999 as being a tri-service *medical surveillance* tool. Also, according to 2004 policy on comprehensive health surveillance, the definition of "medical surveillance" is "the ongoing, systematic collection, analysis, and interpretation of data derived from instances of medical care or medical evaluation, and the reporting of population-based information" (DoDD 6490.02E, para 3.3). The mission obviously drives the types of data that should be collected, analyzed, interpreted, and reported. In order to assess the full range of medical surveillance data requirements, we combed current DoD policy regarding deployment health surveillance and comprehensive health surveillance and formulated the following list:

- instances of disease or injury (DoDD 6490.02E, para 4.4)
- patient encounters—inpatient and outpatient (DoDI 6490.03, para 4.2)
- reportable medical events (DoDI 6490.3, para 4.2)
- medical treatments (DoDD 6490.02E, para 4.4)
- preventive medicines (DoDD 6490.02E, para 4.4)
- immunizations (DoDD 6490.02E, para 4.4)
- deployment location data (DoDI 6490.3, para 4.2)
- lifestyle data (DoDD 6490.02E, para 4.4)
- combat casualties (DoDD 6490.02E, para 4.5.1)
- stress-induced casualties (DoDD 6490.02E, para 4.5.1)
- individual health status (DoDD 6490.02E, para 4.4)
- disease and non-battle injuries (DoDD 6490.02E, para 4.5.1)

According to DoD policy on comprehensive health surveillance, surveillance data must span the entire period of service of military members, and must be transferable to the VA. The data must be timely, and analyses from the data must inform commanders about the health of the force in order to appropriately determine risk and countermeasures. Finally, health surveillance activities must be prioritized based upon the greatest benefit to force health protection planning, response, and decisionmaking (DoDD 6490.02E, paras 4.4 and 4.5).

In addition to the items described in the list above, all captured in DoD policy, the draft AFHSC Concept of Operations (received by RAND on February 29, 2008, after the study had been completed) also specifies that individual medical readiness reporting will now also be encompassed by AFHSC, with the implication that such data would be linked to DMSS. Also, our interviews suggested consideration of additional data elements that are not included in current policy but that could be valuable for medical surveillance and other purposes, e.g., laboratory data from medical records.

DMSS provides a robust database for surveillance data in garrison settings but does not capture all available data elements relevant to deployment surveillance. Table 4.4 provides a detailed comparison of medical surveillance data requirements specified

Table 4.4
Inclusion of Available Medical Surveillance Data in DMSS: Requirements and Opportunities

Type of Data	Garrison Required?	Garrison In DMSS?	Deployment Required?	Deployment In DMSS?
Demographic, administrative	Yes	Yes		
Location	Yes	Yes	Yes	**
Inpatient	Yes	Yes	Yes*	No
Outpatient	Yes	Yes	Yes*	No
Pharmacy	Yes	No	Yes	No
Laboratory	No	No	(N/A)	
Reportable Medical Events	Yes	Yes	Yes	No
Individual Medical Readiness				
Immunizations	Yes	Yes		
Periodic Health Assessment	No	No		
Dental readiness	No	No		
Deployment laboratory tests	No	No		
No deployment limiting condition	No	No		
HIV test result	Yes	Yes		
Casualty	Yes	No		
Deployment health forms	Yes	Yes		
Lifestyle	No	No		

* Includes disease and non-battle injury surveillance.

** Deployment rosters (country level and deployment level) are included in DMSS; specific unit and individual location data are not.

NOTE: Bold border denotes that requirements are not met. Dotted-line border denotes potential opportunities for inclusion in DMSS.

in DoD policy and the data capabilities currently resident in DMSS, in both the garrison and deployment-related context. It also presents a number of available medical surveillance data that are not required but also are not included in the DMSS. The table therefore identifies two kinds of data gaps: those data that are required but not yet included in DMSS (items boxed with heavy lines in the table) and potentially relevant data that are available but not yet incorporated into DMSS (items boxed with dashed lines). The table indicates that most requirements for garrison-based data have been met, whereas most requirements for non-garrison-based data have not. It also suggests available relevant data that, while not required, could be incorporated usefully into DMSS.

As indicated by the table, DMSS is a robust longitudinal surveillance database, particularly for data collected in garrison settings. Much of this information is relevant to deployment health, e.g., the deployment health assessment forms and medical encounters that may follow deployments. In terms of garrison-based data:

- The sources of demographic, administrative, and location characteristics in DMSS (starting at the top of the box in Figure 4.4) are described earlier in this chapter.
- Garrison patient encounter information is generated by DoD's Composite Health Care System and stored by DMSS in the form of Standard Inpatient Data Record files describing inpatient medical diagnostic information and Standard Ambulatory Data Record files for clinical diagnostic information from ambulatory care visits. There are additional data available from such records but not yet linked to DMSS. Clinical and medical record exam data (e.g., vital signs, nurses' notes) are available in the military's electronic medical record systems and are stored in the Military Health System's Clinical Data Repository.
- Information on garrison-based preventive medicines is captured in medical records and pharmacy claims data by AHLTA, the military's current electronic health record, and the Pharmacy Data Transaction Service (PDTS), respectively.
- Laboratory data are not captured in DMSS.
- Reportable medical events in garrison are captured in service-specific systems and fed into DMSS.
- Individual medical readiness indicators (see Chapter Three for further details of this system) are captured and tracked in service data systems, and all but immunization data (which reside in the Defense Enrollment Eligibility Reporting System, or DEERS) are unavailable to DMSS. DEERS data feed into DMSS.
- The HIV test result for a service member is captured by the HIV testing laboratories and is fed into DMSS.
- Casualty information was fed into DMSS through 2003, though it is no longer captured because of security issues.
- Lifestyle factors are captured by service-specific systems, although these are not fed into DMSS.

There are opportunities, nonetheless, to capture more garrison-based data to enrich the medical surveillance and other applications of DMSS, e.g., laboratory data (if these can be standardized sufficiently), additional individual medical readiness indicators, and information related to lifestyle (e.g., behavioral risk factors); most of these are indeed specifically cited by policy as relevant for purposes of medical surveillance. Policy from 1999 specifically calls for the TRICARE Management Activity to provide "unrestricted access to applicable Military Health System data" (ASD(HA), 1999, para 6) for DMSS. The same memorandum also called for DMSS to receive "all theater medical surveillance and treatment data" (para 6). Beyond these medical surveillance data elements are the array of additional occupational and environmental surveillance data (comprising the other piece of "health surveillance"), which are also not captured by DMSS. The draft Concept of Operations for the new AFHSC specifies that such data should ultimately be linked for robust comprehensive health surveillance purposes.

Moreover, measurements of theater-based disease and non-battle injury, reportable medical events, medical treatments, and deployment locations are required in established DoD policy but not currently captured in DMSS. We find for deployment-related data:

- DMSS stores individual country and operation of deployment data for all major CENTCOM deployments since the first Gulf War. However, the location of individuals is not guaranteed from unit-level location data. Detailed individual location data is stored in classified data systems (JMeWS).
- Deployment medical encounter information from a theater of operations—including inpatient, outpatient, and disease and non-battle injury—comes from the Armed Forces Health Longitudinal Technology Application—Theater (AHLTA-T).
- No pharmacy or laboratory data are linked from theater into DMSS.
- In theater, reportable medical events and disease and non-battle injury data are ultimately archived by the JMeWS system. The DNBI system generates daily counts of illness and injury by individual and diagnostic code and aggregates these into broad medical categories determined by the Joint Chiefs of Staff. Yet, we learned from several of our interviewees that the only data fields that are actually classified are those relating to daily locations and not health and DNBI data fields.
- Theater-based casualty information is considered sensitive and is not made available to DMSS.
- Deployment health forms are all sent to AMSA/AFHSC via the services and components, for both the pre- and post-deployment health assessment forms as well as the post-deployment health reassessment form, as described in Chapter Three.

Users and Uses of DMSS

Access to DMSS appeared to be limited to users physically located at AMSA. Written AMSA guidelines and procedures for accessing and general use of DMSS data apparently did not exist. Data within DMSS are obtained from many sources, and some are used subject to the restrictions of various data use agreements, which may be interpreted to restrict the further use or sharing of the data with external customers. According to AMSA analysts, no formal policies were developed or articulated regarding use and access of data sources for which DMSS is the sole custodian (e.g., deployment forms data).

In an article on the DMSS and DoDSR (Rubertone and Brundage, 2002), data access is described as being limited to onsite members of AMSA staff, including AMSA responses to telephonic or written requests for special analyses. According to AMSA analysts, the use of DMSS data by affiliated analysts, under current technical limitations, functionally required co-location of the affiliated analyst with AMSA staff. The Deployment Health Support Directorate, a subdirectorate within the structure of the ASD(HA)'s Force Health Protection and Readiness Division, maintained an onsite analyst who performed queries of DMSS data and who was able to perform analyses of data that reside principally on the ASD(HA) systems by manually transporting the data across facilities. Another affiliated analyst from WRAIR was analyzing mental health data from DMSS.

Specific analyses have been conducted in support of information required to inform policy decisions by the Defense Health Board, Office of the Army Surgeon General, and the Army Proponency Office for Preventive Medicine.

Several of those interviewed outside of AMSA remarked that it was extremely difficult to get data back from DMSS once it was provided by the services, and this situation potentially caused missed opportunities. It must be noted that the ASD(HA) memorandum of 1999 called for data sharing between DMSS and the services.

A wider range of military users can access the more limited derivative online DMED database. Analyses of DMSS data are also available through hard copy and online AMSA (now AFHSC) publications, i.e., the Medical Surveillance Monthly Report. The MSMR provides routine summary analyses of select data captured by DMSS, including monthly updates of deployment health assessments, reportable medical events, febrile respiratory illness in military training centers, and medical conditions of surveillance interest as reported by MTFs. The MSMR also includes reports of recent outbreaks, quarterly force health reports, and other military health related topics of special interest.

Chapter Highlights

To summarize some key findings regarding both DoDSR and DMSS, we found that:

- The main uses of the DoDSR have been for research, and the main users of the repository and data assets have been limited to a relatively small number of DoD and civilian researchers.
- While DoDSR and DMSS have been used for other important purposes such as special HIV surveillance studies, public health investigation, and clinical support, our interviews and analyses suggest the potential for far more robust use, in particular for deployment medical surveillance that includes data from deployed settings, and broader health surveillance (i.e., to include medical and occupational and environmental health surveillance in both garrison and deployment settings).

To summarize some key findings about the serum repository in particular, we found that:

- From 2001 through January 2008, specimens from the DoDSR were requested approximately 120 times.
- The missions of the serum repository as defined by DoD policy include medical surveillance, clinical diagnosis, and epidemiological studies of all illness relating to military service, yet the staff at AMSA perceived its main mission to be one of surveillance.
- The serum repository has a large number of specimens that have become delinked from the individual donor; there is no apparent policy in place to determine how long to store the specimens or what to do with them.
- The repository has no apparent guidelines explaining the decisionmaking process for allowing use of the sera.
- The sera are stored at –30°C rather than at a colder temperature more consistent with current industry standards, e.g., –80°C (a point that becomes more important in our comparison to other repositories).
- Most uses of the repository to date have been for research studies (as opposed to surveillance uses).
- The ability of the sera to support the repository's given missions has not been evaluated since the Armed Forces Epidemiology Board recommendation of 2005 (which recommended archiving of white blood cells for preservation of genetic material), and action has not been taken in response to this recommendation.
- There does not appear to be a mandate for any joint body to routinely and systematically evaluate the value of the sera for surveillance possibilities balancing against resource constraints and emerging threats to the force.

To summarize some key points related to DMSS, we found that:

- There is a disparity between the mission of DMSS as defined in policy and the range of its actual functions. Specifically, the mission of DMSS is to provide tri-service medical surveillance. In order to do this, DMSS needs adequate data elements fed in a timely manner and across a service member's career. DMSS is not currently receiving many relevant data elements, which would be necessary though not necessarily sufficient to address deployment health needs. For example, theater-level data are not being provided to DMSS because of classification issues, in spite of the fact that Congress called on DoD to reexamine the most appropriate level of classification. We have presented other examples of this disparity.

- DMSS was to share data across all services; yet we see no evidence that this is being done except in a very limited way through DMED, and several military interviewees complained about the inadequacy of what they perceive as incomplete DMED data.

- Access seemed to be limited to users physically located at AMSA, although the dataset is unclassified and could ostensibly reside on the NIPRNet. Further, there appear to be no published guidelines explaining why access is limited, to whom it is limited, and so forth.

CHAPTER FIVE

Examination of Other Biological Specimen Repositories

To better evaluate potential improvements to the DoDSR, the RAND team examined the characteristics of other repositories in the United States and abroad. Repositories are typically associated with organizations that have specific research interests or surveillance mandates that necessitate storing of biological specimens. Specific details of each repository are a function of their general purpose, the sponsoring organization, and underlying research design that led to the repository. Depending upon these factors, the collection, processing, testing, and storage of specimens vary across the repositories. The volume and storage conditions of specimens can also be dictated by the purpose and function of the repository.

In the remainder of this chapter, we first describe the different major blood fractions and the types of standard tests that can be performed with them. Then we describe the framework used in this analysis and provide a comparison of key features of the repositories (details about each of the repositories can be found in Appendix C).

Blood Fractions and Testing

As mentioned in Chapter Two, Congress legislated in 1997 that DoD collect blood specimens pre- and post-deployment. Because DoD was already collecting blood for HIV testing and storing sera, it decided to use the extant repository as currently configured to fulfill the newer legal requirement. Since then, both Congress and DoD have questioned the continued use of the repository to fulfill pre- and post-deployment health surveillance functions. The ASD(HA) asked the Armed Forces Epidemiology Board to investigate whether or not other specimens should be stored, and the board concluded that there may be utility in storing white blood cells (for preservation of genetic material).

As described in this section, white blood cells can be either purified and stored as the buffy coat fraction or captured in whole blood; whole blood can be stored either dried or liquid. In all of these cases, DNA and RNA can be captured in adequate amounts for today's technology, and even perhaps tomorrow's, to use in genetic testing.

As further discussed, dried blood spots have several advantages, one being the simplicity of collection, processing, and storage along with the long-term stability of DNA. Whole blood provides buffy coat, which in turn provides even larger amounts of DNA and RNA for genetic testing than do dried blood spots.

Blood is one of the most common biological specimens collected and used for diagnostic tests, and it is also commonly used for surveillance and research purposes. Blood is a complex mixture of cells, proteins, metabolites, and many other substances. Cells make up approximately 45 percent of the total human blood volume. Plasma, the liquid component of blood in which the blood cells are suspended, makes up about 55 percent of total blood volume. Serum is blood plasma without fibrinogen or the other clotting factors. The vast majority of blood cells—more than 99 percent—are erythrocytes (red blood cells, RBC). Thrombocytes (platelets) make up approximately 0.5 percent of cellular blood components, and leukocytes (white blood cells, WBC) make up approximately 0.3 percent. The only human blood cells that contain nuclei and are suitable for use in the preparation of genomic DNA are WBC.

Which specimens are collected, and how they are stored, is often driven by the purpose of the collection or the purpose of the original study that collected the specimens. Depending on the intended use of the specimens, biological repositories store either whole blood or purified blood components (i.e., blood fractions). Whole blood can be collected and stored either in liquid form or as dried blood spots (collection on filter paper). Repositories also store purified fractions from whole blood, which can commonly include serum, plasma, and WBC. During separation, WBC and platelets typically are collected together in a fraction called the buffy coat and are often stored in this form. In some cases, repositories also store RBC.

Blood tests can be grouped into a range of categories, including clinical biochemistry, hematology, immunology, microbiology, and genetic. In general, serum and plasma can both be used for a wide range of biochemistry, immunology, and microbiology tests, although serum is often the preferred fraction, since the clotting factors in plasma can complicate some tests. Plasma is required for blood clotting tests and for some other specific tests like the fasting plasma glucose test for diabetes. Whole blood is required for some hematology tests such as complete blood counts, and it can also be used for a variety of biochemistry, immunology, and microbiology tests.

Genetic-based tests require DNA or RNA, depending on the type of test. This generally requires collection of WBC, either in purified form or in whole blood. Both dried blood spots (DBS) and liquid blood can be used for genetic studies. DBS have long been used for newborn screening and large population-based repositories (Shafer et al., 1996; Hsu et al., 1992)

DBS have the advantage of simpler collection, processing, and storage requirements (–20°C, humidity control, small space requirements) and long-term stability of the DNA (UK Biobank, 2004) but supply a smaller quantity of DNA. Since the size of

DBS specimens is typically small, yielding limited amounts of DNA, they may not be suitable for whole-genome amplification (Steinberg et al., 2002).

The buffy coat from processed whole blood can be stored or further processed to purify specific subsets of WBC, DNA, or RNA. Buffy coat provides more volume of material than DBS for genetic studies. Finally, WBC can be turned into immortal cell lines to provide long-term, high volumes of genetic material. This can be done on freshly purified WBC or on blood properly stored with cryoprotectant in liquid nitrogen.

Framework for Specimen Collection, Processing, Testing, and Storage

To understand and examine the different repositories, the RAND team developed a framework for the collection, processing, testing, and storage of specimens (Figure 5.1). Each of these components includes key variables that affect the usefulness of specimens for different purposes (e.g., research, surveillance). The boxes enclose the overarching elements associated with that component. Each of these components is described in more detail below.

As shown in Figure 5.1, the framework for understanding the characteristics of repositories consists of four components: collection, processing, testing, and storage.

The specimen-collection component of the framework consists of who the specimens are collected from, when and where they are collected, the purpose for which they are collected (i.e., why), and the collection method used (i.e., how). The overarching elements associated with the collection component of the framework are informed consent and institutional review board (IRB) approval. The system of federal protections pertaining to the ethical involvement of people as participants in medical research, including research with biological specimens, involves review of the proposed research by an IRB and a determination of the need for the informed consent of the research participant (see Department of Health and Human Services (HHS) regulations at 45 CFR part 46 and DoD Directive 3216.02).[1] The IRB looks after the participants' rights and the ethics of the research study. The IRB process can vary across institutions and nations, with some countries having a single national board that addresses all research studies involving human participants. IRB approval can be implemented at different

---

[1]   45 CFR part 46 is the Common Rule that addresses the protection of human research participants in the federal government. It is a set of identical regulations codified by 15 agencies, of which DoD is one. (The Office of Science and Technology Policy is a signatory to the Common Rule, but did not codify it because it does not conduct or sponsor research. The Common Rule also regulates research conducted or sponsored by two other agencies that are not signatories but are bound to HHS regulations and therefore the Common Rule: the Social Security Administration and the Central Intelligence Agency.) The Common Rule has to be upheld and is enforceable by law. DoD Directive 3216.02 is the Department of Defense codification of the Common Rule and is equivalent to it.

Figure 5.1
Framework for the Evaluation of Serum Repositories

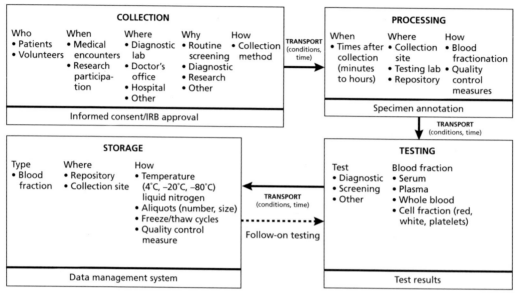

points in the life of a specimen. Most often an initial IRB approval is required prior to the start of a research study, but additional IRB reviews can occur to provide periodical review of the study to ensure that appropriate steps are being taken to protect the participant's rights and welfare. Once specimens are stored in a repository, IRB approval is also usually required for the distribution of specimens for new research studies and to investigators who were not part of the original study. In addition, some repositories have established their own IRBs to oversee access and storage conditions of specimens, as well as other general repository functions.

The specimen-processing component of the framework includes the processing method (e.g., how blood is fractionated), as well as when and where the specimens are processed. Some specimens may need to be transported from the collection site to the laboratory/facility where they will be processed. The overarching element associated with specimen processing is the annotation that accompanies each specimen.

Once the specimen has been processed, testing may be conducted to acquire information about the specimen and the person from whom it came. In some cases, the testing is done at the same facility as the processing; in other cases, testing is done at a different site. The results of tests done on specimens are the overarching element associated with testing.

Finally, once the specimen has been processed and all of the initial testing has been completed, it is put into storage at a biological specimen repository. The storage component of the framework includes the type of specimen being stored, and when, where, and how it is stored. The data management system at a repository is the overarching element associated with storage. The conditions and time involved in the transport processes between collection, processing, testing, and storage introduce additional variables to the framework.

We chose a variety of different repositories that collect blood products to compare with DoDSR, to cover the variables described here.

Six Repositories for Comparison

We collected data from six repositories to compare with the DoDSR. We sought a purposive sample of convenience of repositories that collect, process, and store large numbers of blood specimens, including repositories representing a range of purposes, funding sources, types of blood fractions, and processing and storage conditions. The six repositories are:

- **National Health and Nutrition Examination Survey (NHANES).** A U.S. federally funded biological specimen repository for clinical, epidemiological, and genomic research, drawn from a nationally representative population sample.
- **UK Biobank.** A non-U.S. government- and foundation-funded prospective epidemiological repository designed to include biological specimens and study morbidity and mortality of chronic and other diseases.
- **National Heart, Lung, and Blood Institute (NHLBI).** A U.S. federally funded repository storing specimens from multiple individual research projects;
- **Two U.S. military repositories.** One conducts HIV research (the U.S. Military HIV Research Program Repository at Walter Reed), and one is used for remains identification (DoD DNA Remains Identification Registry at the Armed Forces Institute of Pathology).
- **deCODE.** A private repository designed to develop drugs and diagnostics based on genomic studies of the population of Iceland.

Appendix C summarizes the general characteristics of each repository, including information connected to the framework presented in Figure 5.1. The section below compares the six repositories and DoDSR, and it summarizes the general characteristics across the repositories as well as each one's storage and retrieval conditions.

Comparison of DoDSR and Other Repositories

A comparison of DoDSR with the six repositories chosen for this study revealed some similarities and several differences (see Tables 5.1 and 5.2). NHLBI has been collecting

Table 5.1
Comparison of General Repository Characteristics

	NHANES	UK Biobank	NHLBI	WRAIR: Division of Retrovirology	AFIP: DoD DNA Registry	deCODE	DoDSR
Purpose	Surveillance, research	Research	Research	Research	Forensics/Identification	Research and drug development	Surveillance, investigation, research, clinical support
Population represented	Representative sample of U.S. population	Prospective cohort	Clinical research subjects	Clinical trial subjects	All military service members	Family disease clusters	All military service members
Specimens archived	Plasma, serum, purified DNA	RBC, plasma, serum, buffy coat, purified DNA	Whole blood, plasma, serum, buffy coat, purified DNA	Plasma, serum, buffy coat	Whole blood (dried blood spots)	Whole blood, purified DNA	Serum
Longitudinal specimen collection	No	No*	Study-dependent	Study-dependent	No	No	Yes
Health survey data	Yes	Yes	Yes	Yes	No	Yes	No
Link to medical records	No	Yes	No	No	No	Yes	Yes
Current inventory (2007)	>550,000	~335,000	~3.5 million	~1 million	>5.1 million	>500,000	>43 million
Acquisition rate (per year)	~50,000	~175,000	80,000–130,000	~70,000	~300,000	12,000–60,000	1.9 million
Repository funding	Public (HHS)	Public/Private	Public (HHS)	Public (DoD)	Public (DoD)	Private	Public (DoD)
Informed consent	Yes	Yes	Yes	Yes	Yes	Yes	No
Specimens collected with IRB approval	Yes	Yes	Yes**	Yes	No	Yes	No
Specimens requested for use with IRB approval	Yes	Yes	Yes	Yes	No	Yes	Yes***
Year established	1988****	2001	1975	1986	1992	1998	1989

* UK Biobank does not plan to conduct routine longitudinal sample collection, but does plan to repeat baseline assessments (i.e., questionnaire, measurements, and sample collection) in about 25,000 participants during the recruitment phase and then every 2–3 years during follow-up (UK Biobank, March 21, 2007).

** Also has an additional IRB, conducted through the repository, to address storage of specimens.

*** IRB approval required for research uses.

**** Established in 1956, but storage of specimens started during NHANES III (1988–1994).

Table 5.2
Repository Specimen Storage Characteristics for Blood-Derived Specimens

	NHANES	UK Biobank	NHLBI	WRAIR: Division of Retrovirology	AFIP: DoD DNA Registry	deCODE	DoDSR
Blood fractions							
Whole blood			−80°C / Liq N$_2$			−25°C	
Red blood cells		−80°C / Liq N$_2$					
Plasma	−80°C / Liq N$_2$	−80°C / Liq N$_2$	−80°C / Liq N$_2$	−80°C			
Serum	−80°C / Liq N$_2$	−80°C / Liq N$_2$	−80°C / Liq N$_2$	−80°C			−30°C
Buffy coat		−80°C / Liq N$_2$	−80°C / Liq N$_2$				
Purified DNA	−80°C / Liq N$_2$	−80°C / Liq N$_2$	−80°C / Liq N$_2$	Liq N$_2$		4°C	
Dried blood spots					−20°C		
Retrieval mechanism							
Automated		X				X	
Manual	X	X	X	X	X	X	X

specimens the longest, since 1975, while UK Biobank is the newest repository, having started to collect specimens in 2001. All of the repositories fulfill a research purpose except the AFIP DoD DNA Registry, which is used solely for forensic purposes (i.e., remains identification). DoDSR and NHANES are the only repositories whose purposes include surveillance. All of the repositories are publicly funded except deCODE, which is privately funded; UK Biobank receives both public and private funding. Specifically, DoDSR, WRAIR, and AFIP are funded by DoD.

The number of specimens stored in the repositories ranges from approximately 335,000 specimens at the UK Biobank to more than 43 million specimens at DoDSR. Specimen acquisition rates vary, ranging from approximately 50,000 per year by NHANES to almost 2 million per year by DoDSR. Specimens in the repositories represent different populations; for example, DoDSR and the AFIP DoD DNA Registry contain specimens from all military service members, while NHLBI and WRAIR contain specimens from participants in clinical trials. NHANES contains specimens from a representative sample of the U.S. population of all ages, and the UK Biobank contains a prospective cohort from the U.K. general population aged 40 to 69. deCODE contains specimens representing over half of the adult population of Iceland (i.e., more than 100,000 people). It can employ genealogy to cluster patients affected by any disease into large extended families.[2]

DoDSR only collects serum, which is stored at –30°C; it is the only repository that does not collect DNA or a blood fraction from which DNA could be isolated. AFIP, NHLBI, and deCODE all collect whole blood from which DNA can be isolated. However, each repository stores it differently: AFIP stores whole blood as dried blood spots at –20°C; NHLBI freezes whole blood at –80°C or in liquid nitrogen (storage temperature is study-dependent); and deCODE stores whole blood at –25°C. All of the repositories except AFIP and DoDSR collect more than one blood fraction including purified DNA. NHANES, UK Biobank, NHLBI, and WRAIR store specimens at either –80°C or in liquid nitrogen. All of the repositories use a manual system to retrieve specimens from storage; however, UK Biobank and deCODE also use an automated, robotic retrieval system for some specimens.

DoDSR is the only repository that routinely collects longitudinal specimens; however, both NHLBI and WRAIR have longitudinal specimens from some of the research studies that are included in the repositories. Only DoDSR, UK Biobank, and deCODE currently maintain links to medical records allowing for detailed follow-up of the health of the individuals from whom the samples were obtained. However, all of the repositories except DoDSR and AFIP collect health survey data along with the specimens.

DoDSR is the only repository that does not obtain informed consent from individuals before their specimens are collected. In addition, DoDSR and AFIP are the

---

[2]   For more information see deCODE, "deCODE's Population Approach."

only repositories that collected specimens without prior IRB approval. However, all of the repositories that allow specimens to be used for research purposes require IRB approval; specimens at the AFIP DoD DNA Registry may not be used for research purposes.

As described above and summarized in Tables 5.1 and 5.2, there are a number of important similarities and differences between the DoDSR and other biological repositories. Examination of the purposes, funding sources, and types of blood fractions and their processing and storage across a range of relevant repositories provides an important basis for understanding specimen-related aspects of the current DoDSR and opportunities for potential improvements. We highlight the following comparisons:

- The DoDSR is by far the largest of all the repositories examined here; its total size and annual rate of specimen acquisition are at least ten times those for the civilian repositories described in this chapter.
- The DoDSR has a wide range of purposes, including surveillance, whereas most of the other repositories serve largely research purposes; only NHANES also has a surveillance mission.
- Similar to NHANES (general U.S. population), UK Biobank (general U.K. population) and the AFIP DNA Registry (military population), the DoDSR contains specimens that are statistically representative of a defined population, i.e., beyond a research study population.
- DoDSR, UK Biobank, and deCODE maintain links to medical records; however, only DoDSR routinely collects serial specimens from the same individuals, i.e., longitudinal specimen collection.
- All six of the comparison repositories, but not DoDSR, store blood-derived specimens from which genetic material (DNA or RNA) can be retrieved reliably; storage requirements are different for such specimens (less rigorous temperature requirements for DBS and, in general, colder temperature requirements for all other relevant blood fractions—only deCODE stores whole blood and purified DNA at higher temperatures than the −30°C temperature at which the DoDSR stores its serum specimens).
- Only DoDSR specimens are collected without at least reading an informed consent and privacy statement (even the DoD DNA specimens are collected following reading of these statements); only specimens in the two DoD repositories are collected without prior IRB approval, however, an appropriate IRB must approve use of DoDSR specimens for research purposes.

Chapter Highlights

This chapter lays the groundwork for understanding aspects of the DoDSR related to the specimens themselves and for identifying potential opportunities for improvement based on comparison with a range of other relevant biospecimen repositories. Key points from this chapter include the following:

- As described in this chapter, white blood cells can be either purified and stored as the buffy coat fraction or captured in whole blood; whole blood can be stored either dried or liquid. In all of these cases, DNA and RNA can be captured in adequate amounts for today's technology, and even perhaps tomorrow's, to use in genetic testing.
- Also as we describe here, dried blood spots have several advantages, one being simple collection, processing, and storage along with long-term stability of DNA. Whole blood provides buffy coat, which in turn provides even larger amounts of DNA and RNA for genetic testing than dried blood spots.
- A comparison of the repositories we selected for this study (Table 5.2) shows that the DoDSR is unique in that it stores sera at a relatively warmer temperature than the others, it is the only repository that stores only sera, it is very large compared to the others, and it does not require informed consent. While each of these differences does not indicate that the DoDSR is not meeting the current "best practices" of the industry, it does indicate that DoD has opportunities to address each of these issues within its unique context to deliberately assess whether or not it is functioning as intended. The DoDSR will soon be forced to consider how it is going to acquire more space, and as we discuss in the next chapter, this presents an opportunity for DoD to determine whether or not changes are warranted.

CHAPTER SIX

Identification of Potential Improvement Strategies

In this chapter we present the main findings from our analyses and potential improvement strategies. This discussion draws upon our analysis of the material covered to this point in the report, including document review and interviews with key military and civilian experts, and it is organized based on the conceptual framework first described in Chapter One and presented again here as Figure 6.1.

We present our findings and then identify and assess potential improvement strategies, grouped according to the various domains of the framework. For each, we summarize relevant current characteristics of the DoDSR-DMSS system (described in greater detail elsewhere in this report), describe findings (often issues or problems) derived from our analyses and key informant interviews, and finally present potential

Figure 6.1
Conceptual Framework to Help Identify Potential Improvements to System Elements

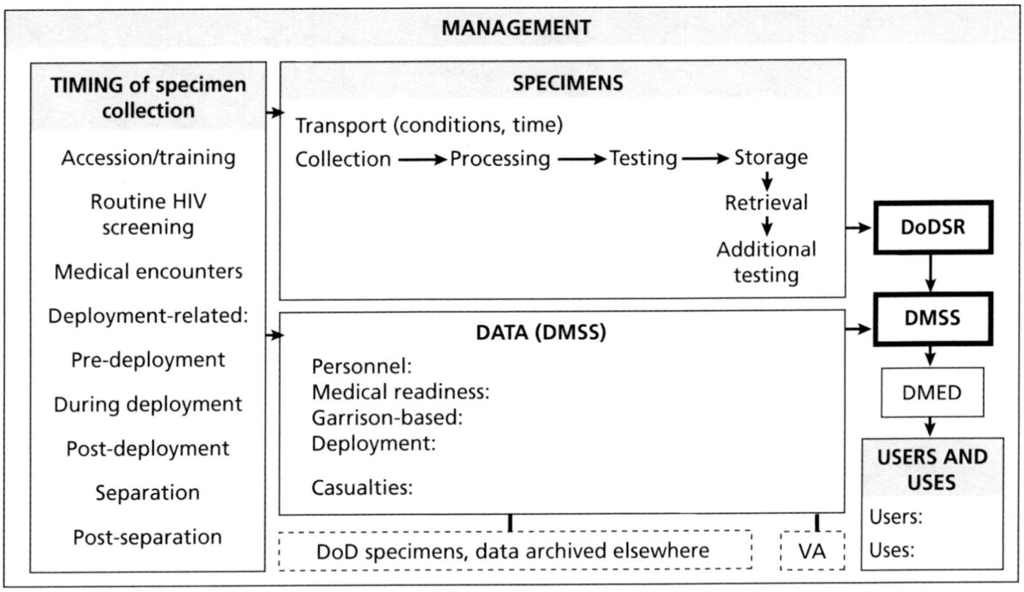

RAND *MG875-6.1*

strategies to address relevant findings. Potential improvements are described in terms of the questions to be addressed, strategies to address them, approach to implementation, and potential advantages and disadvantages. In Chapter Seven, we package the most promising strategies into practical recommendations for action.

Here we present our discussion of issues raised by the current system and potential improvement opportunities. Current system characteristics, as described in detail in Chapter Four, and issues raised about them during our interviews, are summarized in the discussions that follow and in Figure 6.2, which represents a populated version of the conceptual framework shown in Figure 6.1, depicting the current characteristics of the DoDSR-DMSS system. The sections that follow describe our findings and potential improvement strategies. Those strategies are summarized in Figure 6.3, presented at the end of the chapter.

Management

Current Status

Until late February 2008, AMSA was the designated executive agent for military health surveillance (DoDD 6490.3) and as such was the U.S. military's central epidemio-

Figure 6.2
Summary of Current DoDSR/DMSS System Elements and Characteristics

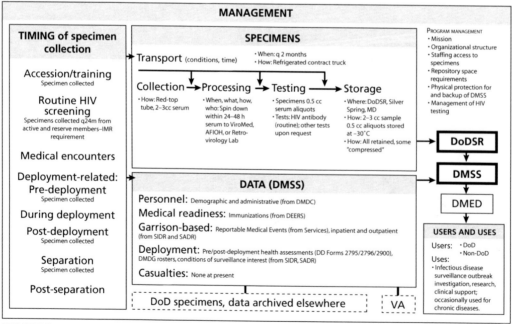

logical resource. AMSA's responsibilities are now subsumed under the new AFHSC. AMSA managed the DoDSR and DMSS systems and the associated DMED database that can be accessed by military users outside of AMSA/AFHSC. Consistent with AMSA's own guidelines (from 2003, still referenced on the new AFHSC web site as of August 2008), access to repository specimens was ultimately the decision of the AMSA director. AMSA's guidelines provide information about submitting requests, but do not address the precise decisionmaking process. Under current institutional requirements, specimens are housed in leased space in Silver Spring, Maryland (lease expires in 2010). The 25,000-square-foot facility accommodates the current inventory of approximately 43 million specimens, some of which have been reconfigured into "compressed" space due to storage space limitations and are thus less readily accessible.

Findings

AMSA's mission statement did not capture explicitly all core functions. In interviews, AMSA staff and leadership frequently alluded to their surveillance mission, suggesting it was the sole, or at least primary, mission for which they were resourced. However, the AMSA mission statement described very general surveillance activities without using the term "surveillance" or referring to "deployment surveillance":

> The Army Medical Surveillance Activity's (AMSA) main functions are to analyze, interpret, and disseminate information regarding the status, trends, and determinants of the health and fitness of U.S. military (and military-associated) populations and to identify and evaluate obstacles to medical readiness. AMSA is the central epidemiological resource for the U.S. Armed Forces providing regularly scheduled and customer-requested analyses and reports to policy makers, medical planners, and researchers. It identifies and evaluates obstacles to medical readiness by linking various databases that communicate information relevant to service members' experience that has the potential to affect their health. (AMSA Mission, personal correspondence, January 28, 2008)

DoD policy has defined a broader set of mission areas for DMSS and DoDSR: medical and deployment health surveillance, including clinical diagnosis and epidemiological studies (DoDD 6490.02E), and deployment-related data (from both garrison and deployed settings) for DoD-wide surveillance and research (ASD(HA), September 30, 1999). Thus, policy seems to suggest that AMSA, as previous executive agent for DMSS and DoDSR (a responsibility now assigned to the new AFHSC), must support the missions of not only medical and deployment health surveillance but also clinical management, epidemiologic investigations, and research toward development of measures for the "prevention and control of diseases associated with military service" (DoDD 6490.02E). Although AMSA's mission statement did not refer explicitly to "deployment health surveillance" or even "surveillance," AMSA's 2003 "Guidelines for Collecting, Maintaining, Requesting, and Using Specimens Stored in the Department of Defense Serum Repository" (still referenced on the AFHSC web site as of August 2008) reflects the full range of mission areas with the exception of "deployment health" as a category for use of requested serum specimens.

It is important to note that CHPPM does not have the lead responsibility for research within the Army. That lies with the Medical Research and Materiel Command (MRMC), which is responsible for medical research, development, and acquisition; medical information management and information technology; medical logistics management; and health facility planning. MRMC is headquartered at Fort Detrick, Maryland, and supports 14 laboratories and separate organizations throughout the United States. Six of the MRMC medical laboratories and institutes perform core science and technology research specializing in infectious diseases, combat casualty care, operational medicine, and chemical and biological defense. The military infectious disease research program focuses on vaccine development against diseases that threaten military personnel, prophylactic and treatment drugs for infectious diseases, techniques for identification of disease organisms and diagnosis of disease, studies of vector controls, and collection of epidemiological data relevant to disease. Thus, while serum specimens stored in the DoDSR and managed by AMSA/AFHSC within CHPPM are relevant to military research, the research function itself is managed by a separate command, MRMC.

Analysis of our interviews suggests that there is a lack of shared understanding within the Army and across DoD of both the mission and appropriate uses of the repository. Some interviewees felt that there is no explicit vision for the repository, perhaps reflecting the lack of common understanding of its full range of missions. There is also a lack of common understanding of the meaning of such missions/terms as "surveillance" and "research." To our knowledge, critical nuances related to the definition and allowable scope of "medical surveillance" and "research" have not been clarified by central (or even Army) guidance. However, AMSA's 2003 guidelines do begin to tease this out, distinguishing between "research" and "nonresearch" studies. Thus the specific research mission for DMSS and DoDSR may present a source of conflict for AMSA (now AFHSC), fundamentally a surveillance entity, yet the designated executive agent for DoDSR and DMSS programs that serve mission areas beyond surveillance alone, including research. Thus, to the extent that DoDSR and DMSS are used for research purposes, AMSA/AFHSC must have at least a research support mission, and the connections between research policy components, e.g., MRMC, and AMSA/AFHSC, must be reconciled.

This confusion plays out in the management of the serum repository. The DoDSR has a set of published guidelines, which define research as studies with

the primary intention to create, extend, or validate generalizable knowledge—that is, knowledge that applies to individuals, populations, or settings external to and not directly associated with the donors of specimens from which the knowledge is generated. (DoDSR, 2003, p. 7)

"Nonresearch" is defined as studies that are specific to identified individuals or populations or settings that those populations represent. The same guidelines signal that nonresearch study requests will be responded to "more quickly" than research, indicating some sort of prioritizing (DoDSR, 2003, p. 7). AMSA's definition of "nonresearch" studies may help legitimize work undertaken by its own staff in response to requests for DMSS data analyses; even so, there are true "research" studies that have also made good use of DMSS data and/or DoDSR specimens (see Chapter Four). Our analyses, validated by interviews, suggest that explicit clarification and prioritization of the range of uses for the DoDSR, and priorities for AMSA/AFHSC staff support, could be helpful to deconflict the range of uses that may go beyond AMSA/AFHSC's designated core surveillance mission, function, and funding stream.

AMSA's organizational position and mission potentially limit use of the repository. AMSA was buried deep within the Army's Medical Command and had a strictly surveillance mission. Its surveillance mission may have limited the broader use of serum specimens, i.e., for purposes beyond surveillance (for which serum specimens are of limited value, at least in real time). Moreover, some interviewees commented on the organization and leadership of AMSA as potentially limiting optimum use of the repository. Interviewees expressed hope that creation of the new AFHSC will offer opportunities to overcome real or perceived organizational factors that may have impeded robust use of DoDSR and/or DMSS in the past.

Small staffing size may have challenged AMSA's ability to fulfill even its primary surveillance mission. Requests for support to other mission areas also put pressure on AMSA's limited staff. AMSA staffing comprised mainly Army and civilian personnel. Also, according to AMSA, the deployments of at least three of its military staff in recent years caused more frequent staff turnover than usual, leading some AMSA staff to comment on issues of staffing strategies, e.g., longer-term billets or more civilian staffing, that might better serve institutional continuity. Finally, the almost exclusive military staffing by Army personnel raised questions among some interviewees about the true tri-service nature of AMSA and the DoDSR-DMSS system it oversees; some contrasted AMSA to GEIS, whose staffing was often perceived as more diverse across services. The creation of the AFHSC in early 2008, with responsibility for both of these programs, offers opportunities to improve the tri-service nature of the DoDSR-DMSS resources.

Transparency in access to specimens may be an issue. DoDI 6490.03 calls for the Secretary of the Army to "establish procedures to respond to requests" for data and specimens. Our main source of information about operational access to DoDSR specimens came from interviews with key informants. While some interviewees noted that they had had no problems in accessing repository specimens, others expressed concern about what they perceived as difficult access or lack of transparent procedures. AMSA, for its part, was open to considering a new mechanism to improve oversight of the approval process for release of specimens. In addition, AMSA staff noted concerns that time-sensitive requests for specimens could not be met consistently, for example if recent pre-deployment specimens needed for an ongoing outbreak investigation have not yet arrived at the repository.

The mixing of uses and long-term storage of specimens, without apparent communication to donors, could be problematic for human subjects protection. The protection of human subjects with regard to the serum repository generally involves two practices: the use of an IRB, and the gaining of informed consent, where appropriate, from service members. We have described in detail the intricacies of both practices as they relate to the collection, storage, and research or nonresearch use of stored sera (see Chapter Four). One of the key issues is that specimens are drawn for either HIV testing or pre- and post-deployment surveillance, and then later could potentially be used for research, patient care, public health/force health protection, and even criminal investigations. Related to this, the sera are stored in perpetuity, and there appears to be no explicit communication of this to the individuals donating them. The mixing of uses and the enduring storage of the specimens, all with no apparent communication to the donors, could be problematic in terms of human subjects protections. Finally, the 2003 AMSA guidelines (still in place, based on the AFHSC web site as of August 2008) that describe the various practices pertaining to each type of use of the sera are not explicit in all cases about whether consent is needed or even whether an IRB is needed.

The current repository facility is not sufficient to support future growth. Approximately 43 million specimens have accumulated over the years. Of those, approximately 5.5 million cannot be linked to records in DMSS, and most of these unlinked specimens have been placed in "compressed" configuration in response to growing limitations in repository storage space. The current repository facility does not provide sufficient space for further growth. At present, no specimens are discarded. AMSA staff noted that selective culling of such specimens would be tedious and not necessarily result in major gains in storage space, since sera are stored in boxes with multiple specimens each. Potential culling of older specimens was called into question by other interviewees, who described the value of military serum specimens from the 1950s–1960s, stored elsewhere, that had been very useful in studying the emergence of hepatitis C. In any case, the upcoming relocation of the repository once the current lease expires provides a timely opportunity to consider space (and other repository) requirements into the future.

The DMSS physical infrastructure and lack of backup pose a risk of system malfunction or failure. The facility used to house the DMSS hardware and operations center was characterized by AMSA analysts as not meeting industry standards and as containing vulnerabilities posing serious risk to system malfunction or failure, such as leaks in the roof of the room housing the DMSS server. A weather incident in late January 2008 involving the DMSS server emphasized the need for both physical protection of DMSS hardware and facilities and robust backup mechanisms for the DMSS database itself.

Some AMSA interviewees commented on the fragmented nature of HIV testing. HIV testing is conducted at different laboratories across the services: by AFIOH, the Army retrovirology laboratory at WRAIR, and ViroMed. Despite comments about fragmentation of testing, we found no evidence that this poses a problem, and no interviewee expressed dissatisfaction with the performance of any of these laboratories.

Potential Improvement Strategies

Based on the problems identified, there are several key questions related to aspects of program management:

- Could the use of DoDSR-DMSS be improved through a clarification or redefinition of the mission of AMSA/AFHSC and DoDSR-DMSS, the new AFHSC organizational structure itself, a different size or skill set of AMSA/AFHSC staff, and/or different procedures for accessing serum specimens or data?
- Given the current storage space constraints, what requirements for space should be sought for the new repository facility following expiration of the current lease? Should archived specimens be selectively culled?
- What improvements can or should be made to current DMSS operating facilities and hardware, given the risks posed by the poor condition of the facilities that house the system?
- Should HIV testing be consolidated within DoD?

The following strategies address these questions.

Strategy 1: Clarify or redefine the mission of AMSA/AFHSC and appropriate uses of the DoDSR, and define relevant terms clearly.

This strategy involves clarification by appropriate military authorities of the scope of "surveillance" and "research" functions, the full range of missions authorized for DMSS and DoDSR, and implications for their executive agent, previously AMSA and now AFHSC. Does the mission of AFHSC itself need to be more explicit to include medical surveillance and deployment health surveillance (including near-real-time medical surveillance from deployment areas), and should it also explicitly include support to clinical management, epidemiological investigations, and research? Or was AMSA's mission of DoDSR and DMSS oversight sufficient to support other DoD entities in these additional mission areas?

After clarification at the policy level, this information should be shared widely and incorporated into practice by AMSA/AFHSC and its chain of command, and shared with all current and potential users of DMSS and DoDSR DoD-wide. This strategy may or may not require new policy/doctrine in and of itself, but the creation of the new AFHSC and attendant requirements for updating relevant DoD policy offers opportunities to be more explicit in describing and aligning the missions of DoDSR, DMSS, and their oversight organization, the new AFHSC. Communications will also require leadership to help assure clearer common understanding across DoD of the full roles and responsibilities of AFHSC, DMSS, and DoDSR, which in turn should lead to more robust and efficient use of these important military resources. There appear to be few if any disadvantages, other than to note that supporting a functionally expanded set of missions may require additional staffing, discussed below in Strategy 3. Perhaps AMSA's 2003 guidelines distinguishing between "research" and "nonresearch" studies using DoDSR specimens were aimed at least in part at reconciling their support to "research" studies, as well as potential human subjects protection issues.

Strategy 2: Change the organizational structure and provide strong leadership.

In late February 2008 the Deputy Secretary of Defense issued a memorandum officially establishing AFHSC, consolidating AMSA and GEIS within an elevated single organizational unit whose director reports directly to the CHPPM Commanding General. The final structure of the organization is to become tri-service. This is an effort to further integrate military health surveillance, in terms of bringing together the complementary functions both of AMSA and GEIS and of other surveillance organizations. Broad experience with organizational restructuring, however, suggests that reorganization alone will likely not be sufficient to fully integrate surveillance and optimize use of the DoDSR-DMSS resources. Also needed are continued strong leadership, efforts to attract strong multiservice military staff, and efforts to create normative change across the military in which the new AFHSC helps the DoDSR-DMSS achieve its full potential through clear mission and successful implementation perceived as timely and helpful by users. Further, as technology advances and the needs of the services change, the AFHSC could play an ongoing oversight and monitoring role to manage a process to determine when relevant new technologies, such as those for collecting, processing, testing, and storing biological specimens, are ripe enough for practical use in the services.

Strategy 3: Align staffing with mission.

Expansion of the mission or uses of the DoDSR-DMSS resources may require changes in the staffing pattern, e.g., in terms of size and skill mix or expansion of relevant contracts, most notably the data analysis contracts. Beyond adding billets to AFHSC's staff or resources to its contracts, there may be low-cost ways to augment staffing, such as offering rotations to military Preventive Medicine Residents and/or epidemiology students from Uniformed Services University of the Health Sciences. Regardless of change in mission, however, drawing its highly qualified professional staff from across all services (as GEIS has done, for example) may contribute to the positive perception and enhanced use of the repository across DoD. There may also be a role for longer military tours for analysts and/or civilian staffing of relevant staff or leadership positions (e.g., deputy director) to optimize institutional continuity.

Strategy 4: Improve transparency in access to specimens.

The most reasonable approach to implementation of this strategy is probably a consensus planning effort culminating in doctrine disseminated across DoD. As a practical matter, this could involve revision and reissuance of the 2003 AMSA guidelines, to add criteria for release of repository specimens, or issuance of a separate document with this information. Further, based on suggestions from various interviewees, such procedures should also include an administrative fast-track mechanism for approval and release of specimens needed on a time-sensitive basis, such as investigation of an ongoing outbreak or for urgent clinical support. Such procedures should be thoroughly vetted, captured in appropriate doctrine, disseminated widely, and followed in practice.

Strategy 5: Improve internal oversight of DoDSR specimen release.

In its April 2005 memorandum the Armed Forces Epidemiology Board (AFEB) recommended consideration of "the creation of an oversight panel to help govern access to the archived specimens," but we could find no evidence that this recommendation was acted upon. Oversight of human subject protections is particularly important if the use of repository specimens expands significantly beyond the original intended uses, e.g., research or other uses judged to require informed consent. During our interviews, AMSA in particular expressed interest in an appropriately constituted group to help oversee the approval of release of repository specimens as well as independent (of service IRB's) oversight of ethical/human subjects issues relevant to the repository. The new AFHSC may wish to consider establishing its own IRB if it is felt that an additional layer of human subjects review is warranted. In addition to IRB review, the U.S. National Heart, Lung, and Blood Institute (NHLBI) has constituted an allocation committee that reviews requests for specimens (see Chapter Five). This allocation committee may provide a relevant model to AFHSC for dealing with requests for serum specimens.

Strategy 6: Collect specimens with informed consent.

The 2003 AMSA guidelines, still in force as of August 2008, are not explicit about all cases when consent may or may not be required. In the cases when consent is not required, guidelines specify that the specimens be "delinked" from individually identifying information. Currently, and consistent with the waiver provision in existing legislation on privacy protection and informed consent, specimens stored in DoDSR are collected without informed consent. For that reason, in part, specimens that are sent to researchers for research purposes are delinked from any identifiable information. This also limits the utility of the specimens in the repository, since there is no way for researchers to request more of the same specimen, and it restricts research to strictly retrospective studies, since it is not possible to obtain specimens from the same individual in the future once it has been delinked from identifiable information.

Sera are drawn for either HIV testing or pre- and post-deployment surveillance, but they can be used for other purposes and are stored in perpetuity. None of this is apparently explained to service members. As concerns about protecting the privacy of human subjects continue to be raised, and to broaden the usefulness of the specimens in the repository, DoDSR should consider obtaining informed consent for the storage and research use of specimens in DoDSR.

Also, the DoDSR is charged with the storage of specimens from service members and civilians in the military community. The 2003 AMSA guidelines do not address the use of an IRB in all described cases of use, and when they do they rely on the IRB approval of the requesting agency. There is a trend among repositories to either have an internal IRB or to be closely affiliated with an outside IRB. Therefore, AMSA may wish to pursue a strategy to establish its own IRB for the DoDSR or become affiliated with a tri-service IRB that would protect not only service members' interests, but ensure that protocols take into consideration the protection of the Military Health System and the DoDSR while still allowing for the conduct of appropriate research and nonresearch.

Strategy 7: Determine requirements for the new repository.

Once any modifications are made to plans for future collection and/or archiving of specimens, planners must determine the time horizon and associated requirements for space in the new repository facility. For example, if the current 25,000-square-foot repository accommodates approximately 43 million specimens, with some redundancy to mitigate potential equipment failure, and with an acquisition rate of approximately 1.9 million new specimens per year, then a new repository configured similarly but with double the capacity should suffice for the next 23 years. However, if specimens are to be collected more frequently or for an extended period of time, e.g., following separation, then space requirements and planning horizon must take these new requirements into account. This is a timely juncture for undertaking such planning, however, since the current repository lease expires in 2010, and any new space requirements must be established soon.

Strategy 8: Protect the physical infrastructure and back up DMSS.

An incident in late January 2008 involving a DMSS server emphasized the potential vulnerabilities of both the facility housing the DMSS operation as well as the system hardware on which the DMSS system currently operates. An in-depth assessment of the current facility and potential risks posed by the physical state of the facility should be undertaken. At the very least, planning requirements for the new AFHSC facility should provide for adequate housing and protection of the integrity of the database itself. Offsite backup systems as well as data mirroring are important ways to secure the continuity of DMSS operations and maintain the integrity and utility of service member information. Securing the maintenance and integrity of DMSS data is paramount to AFHSC's ability to meet its stated mission objectives and continue to support military health in a consistent and reliable manner.

Strategy 9: Consider consolidation of HIV testing.

From a systems perspective, DoD could consider potential efficiencies to be gained by consolidating HIV screening in a single (e.g., military or contract) laboratory. However, our analyses did not yield compelling justification for this strategy.

At present, the laboratory with the highest throughput capacity is that of AFIOH; and at present the WRAIR HIV laboratory currently performs all HIV testing for the European Command. Under Base Realignment and Closure plans, AFIOH is scheduled to be relocated to Wright-Patterson AFB in Ohio. Several of those interviewed across the services commented on the potential desirability of co-locating the laboratory and the repository, including the possibility of establishing a new laboratory for purposes of HIV screening and potentially other testing. Another option would be to co-locate the AFIOH laboratory and new serum repository, whether at the new AFIOH site in Ohio or the new repository site in the National Capital Region (where the new AHFSC will also reside). If any co-location strategy is to be seriously considered, decisions should be made relatively soon—since both AFIOH and the serum repository facility will be relocated within the next few years. Further, any benefits in either co-location of the laboratory and repository or consolidation of HIV screening in a single military laboratory (e.g., potential cost savings, improved management efficiency, increased military laboratory surge capacity) should be weighed against the costs and administrative requirements associated with deviations from current plans. Military leadership will likely wish to make any relevant planning decisions within the near-term planning frame for the new AFIOH and repository facilities.

Timing of Specimen Collection

Current Status

In general, blood specimens are collected according to administrative milestones. Specimens are routinely collected and archived at accession, pre- and post-deployment, and at separation, as well as every two years for HIV screening. No specimens collected from routine medical encounters, during deployments, or post-separation are archived.

Findings

The current frequency and timing of specimen collection from service members appears to be adequate. In 2005 the Armed Forces Epidemiology Board (now the Defense Health Board) endorsed continuation of the universal sampling and current timing of pre- and post-deployment specimen collection. Most of our military interviewees did not see good reason to collect routine HIV specimens more frequently or on dates tagged to birth month, nor to collect and archive additional specimens from routine medical encounters (other than those from which specimens are already required) or theater operations.

There are divergent views regarding the desirability of ongoing specimen collection from separated members enrolled in the VA health system. This group represents an estimated 8 million of the approximately 25 million eligible. According to the VA, such individuals tend to remain within the VA health care system for life, thus extending the longitudinal coverage of service members for years or decades beyond their active duty. Policymakers in OSD and the VA expressed strong support for extending the period of longitudinal serum and data collection beyond separation, while at least one AMSA staff member expressed reservations, seemingly based on perceived administrative complexity. AMSA did suggest, however, that they would be supportive of continued specimen collection from separated military members treated at MTFs. Because our study was completed before AFHSC was created, we are unaware of AFHSC's views on this matter.

Potential Improvement Strategy

Based on our findings, the one key question related to the timing of specimen collection concerns the extension of collection beyond active duty:

- Is there justifiable benefit in extending specimen collection from separated service members followed in MTFs and/or the VA health system?

The following strategy addresses this question.

Strategy 10: Extend routine specimen collection beyond separation.

Two implementation options, not mutually exclusive, include extending systematic specimen collection on a voluntary basis from separated military members followed at MTFs—an estimated 2 million members separated from active duty currently enrolled in TRICARE Prime or eligible for TRICARE for Life combined (DoD Task Force, December 20, 2007) and doing the same for the even larger group of separated service members followed by the VA health system—estimated 8 million currently enrolled (CBO, December 2007). A decision on this strategy should be made relatively soon, however, so that planning for the new repository space can accommodate any new space requirements. It is also possible that specimens collected through the VA

system could be archived elsewhere, e.g., through the VA, but in any case both specimens and data collected by the VA and MTFs should be linked to DMSS to assure
the seamless longitudinal nature of data and specimens from service members through
their years of active duty and post-separation. If such a strategy is contemplated, DoD
should also consider the epidemiologic value of a self-selected cohort as compared to
more methodologically rigorous establishment of cohorts of separated service members, which would be considerably more complicated from a practical point of view.

Specimens

Current Status

Currently, specimens that ultimately reach the repository are collected in a single tube
and usually processed within 24–48 hours of collection. Shelf time before initial processing may vary depending on individual versus mass specimen collection. Serum
is extracted and tested for HIV. Initial HIV testing is performed by ViroMed (the
laboratory contractor for U.S.-based Army and Navy/Marine specimens), AFIOH (for
all Air Force specimens), or the Army's retrovirology laboratory at WRAIR (for specimens coming from Europe). The Army and Navy/Marines have separate contracting
processes, but currently both employ ViroMed. Serum remaining after HIV screening,
usually about 2–3cc, is sent to the repository. Shipping temperature requirements are
in place, but they are not rigorously monitored.

The transport contractor picks up specimens approximately every two months
from the ViroMed in Minnesota and from AFIOH in Texas and then transports them
in a freezer truck to the repository in Maryland. Specimens are shipped and stored
frozen in walk-in freezers maintained at –30°C. Specimens are retrieved manually
from the walk-in freezers. Upon first request for a specimen from the repository, there
is a single freeze-thaw cycle for aliquoting. The specimen is thawed, divided into multiple 0.5cc aliquots, and then used for further analyses or frozen and stored at –30°C
until it is needed. Serum specimens are released as 0.5cc aliquots to approved users for
approved testing purposes.

Findings

Variations exist in specimen processing and transport conditions. There are significant variations and a lack of standardization in the length of time that specimens
sit at the MTF before being processed (i.e., spun down) to obtain serum, and the transport time (24–48 hours) of serum from the MTF to the testing laboratory. In addition,
several interviewees, from both AMSA and across military services, commented on
problems of timeliness in the repository's receiving recently obtained specimens, e.g.,
accession or pre-deployment specimens needed for investigation of outbreaks. The two-

monthly schedule for transport of specimens to the repository contributes to delays in the accessibility of such specimens, e.g., to support real-time outbreak investigations.

The finite size of the archived serum specimens limits the number of uses from a single specimen. The current 0.5cc aliquot size means that a given 2–3cc serum specimen can only be used 4–6 times. The RAND team identified this as a possible issue, and a number of interviewees also expressed concern.

At DoDSR, storing the specimens in 2–3cc vials requires a freeze-thaw cycle before the specimen reaches the end user. Freezing and thawing biological specimens can impact the measurement of many components of the specimen, including biomarkers and genetic material. Some other repository models minimize the freeze-thaw cycles of their specimens.

Archiving of other blood fractions might be desirable. The RAND team was explicitly asked to consider whether blood-derived specimens other than serum should be archived. Indeed, in 2005 the Armed Forces Epidemiology Board recommended the preservation of WBC for this purpose, but there has been no apparent action on that recommendation. There are clearly considerations related to policy, logistics, and cost associated with any such change. For example, dried whole blood spots offer promising opportunities to retain genetic material and are associated with only modest requirements for space and storage conditions. The inclusion of new types of specimen in the repository would most certainly mean different storage requirements and perhaps also different retrieval processes, both of which should be considered in light of the anticipated relocation of the repository. As part of our data collection on this question, we also solicited the views of key informants. Most of the specimen-related discussions with interviewees focused on the utility of serum specimens as currently stored and the desirability—or not—of archiving other blood-derived specimens, most notably fractions that would retain adequate genetic material. Several interviewees expressed interest in collecting dried whole blood spots on filter paper.

If new types of specimens are contemplated, alternate storage conditions must also be considered. The current repository stores serum specimens at −30° C, which also permits the use of large walk-in freezers. If new types of specimens or different storage conditions for serum specimens are contemplated, associated new requirements must also be considered, as AFHSC secures a new repository facility within the next several years. For example, storage at a colder temperature such as −80°C would not permit walk-in freezers.

Current routine screening is limited to HIV. Some AMSA interviewees raised the possibility of running a routine panel of tests on serum specimens before they are (re)frozen and stored. Neither DoD policy nor other key informants explicitly indicate requirements or current needs for additional routine screening, and there are clearly both logistical and resource issues if additional routine screening is to be considered.

Potential Improvement Strategies

Based on our findings, the key questions related to blood specimens concern the cold chain maintenance of specimens, timeliness of transport to the repository, finite size of archived sera, number of required freeze-thaw cycles, the potential for other routine screening tests, the desirability of retaining additional blood fractions that would permit a wider range of testing, and storage temperature of the specimens:

- How could the cold chain be monitored better?
- How can accessibility to recently collected specimens be improved?
- Given that it is almost certainly impractical to collect and store larger specimens (greater volume of serum), should smaller aliquots be considered?
- Can the number of freeze-thaw cycles be reduced, as another way to preserve testable analytes in the specimens?
- Should new routine screening tests be added?
- Should additional blood fractions be retained, and if so, are potential new requirements justified?
- Should specimens from other studies be archived in the central repository, or at least be accessible through links into DMSS?

The following strategies address these questions.

Strategy 11: Improve the cold chain custody of specimens.

Specimens are collected throughout the country and world at MTFs, clinics, hospitals, etc. and shipped to AFIOH, WRAIR HIV laboratory, or ViroMed for testing. However, laboratory personnel do not have adequate cold chain custody for specimens. There is no way to determine whether the specimens were maintained at controlled temperatures before arrival at the testing facility. There are simple devices that can track the temperature of a shipment continuously or track the highest temperature that a package reached during transit. Either of these options would allow laboratory personnel to know whether the specimens have been compromised by reaching high temperature levels. Once tested, specimens from AFIOH and ViroMed are frozen and shipped to the repository in a refrigerated truck. Specimens from WRAIR HIV laboratory are delivered to DoDSR weekly on dry ice. It would also be useful to maintain records of the refrigerated truck temperature as AFIOH and ViroMed specimens are being transported.

Strategy 12: Increase the frequency of specimen shipment to the repository.

Increasing the frequency of specimen shipment, e.g., from the current two-monthly schedule to monthly, could be achieved through modification of the current specimen transport contract or purchase of a vehicle for this purpose. While we understand that a vehicle was recently purchased for this purpose, we are not sure if this is actually the case and that specimen shipments are now more frequent; we therefore decided to include this strategy. Either option, i.e., more frequent transport by the contractor or purchase of a truck for specimen transport, increases the cost to the military, either one-time or recurring. However, more timely archiving of specimens can potentially render the repository more relevant for real-time support of serosurveillance, investigations, and clinical management. If this remains an issue, AFHSC should consider the most desirable timing and efficient mechanism for transport of specimens to the repository. In lieu of more frequent shipments, another option would be to develop a policy to allow expedited shipment of specimens from the testing laboratories for special circumstances when specimens are needed quickly.

Strategy 13: Reduce the number of routine freeze-thaw cycles.

The measurement of biomarkers in blood specimens has become an integral component of many epidemiologic studies. As noted above, freezing and thawing biological specimens can affect the measurement of many components of the specimen, including biomarkers and genetic material (Mitchella et al., 2005). Most repositories and researchers minimize the number of times a specimen is frozen and thawed. In addition, NHANES takes part of its specimens and freezes aliquots in liquid nitrogen to save as a pristine specimen. DoDSR procedures could change to provide for aliquoting the specimens before they are frozen and shipped to the storage facility. This would increase costs associated with storage and shipping.

Strategy 14: Reduce the size/volume of serum aliquots released for testing.

With current testing methods, the volume of specimens required for testing has been reduced, although it varies by analyte and test protocol. Currently DoDSR sends all requestors a 0.5cc aliquot. For many tests, a smaller volume would be sufficient. For instance, aliquots of 0.25cc would double the number of specimens available from an individual specimen. For rare cases that 0.5cc aliquots are actually required, two vials could be sent. However, the issue of running out of specimens has not been a problem with the repository to date, and will only be an issue if DoDSR significantly increases the number of specimens that are provided to researchers and other users. However, increasing the number of aliquots by decreasing their size may require additional storage space.

Strategy 15: Perform a standard set of tests on serum specimens.

If AFHSC wants to be more proactive in performing surveillance with the specimens in the DoDSR, a set of predetermined tests could be performed on all, or subsets of, the specimens as they are collected. This would allow AFHSC personnel to perform more immediate surveillance activities. Other repositories, such as NHANES, perform a standard set of biological tests on the blood specimens they collect, and the results of these tests are then made available to researchers who request data and specimens. In addition, those researchers are often required to submit the results of their tests back to the repository, which then become part of the data available to other researchers. This strategy would require new laboratory and/or financial resources to support a new routine panel of tests. It is not clear that all potentially worthwhile routine tests could be identified in advance, nor whether they would remain constant over time. The advantages of this strategy would be the availability of more routine test results from each specimen (or selected specimens) from which to perform routine surveillance and a reduction in the freeze-thaw cycles before having such results. The disadvantages relate mostly to resources: financial, human, and laboratory. Nonetheless, it may be worthwhile to ask an appropriately constituted military body to consider this question in more detail, to identify potentially useful tests and specific advantages and disadvantages, and then to weigh these carefully and offer recommendations.

Strategy 16: Collect and archive blood fractions that permit a wider range of testing.

Other repositories collect and store a wider range of specimens including whole blood, plasma, serum, white blood cells (often as buffy coat), and purified DNA specimens. While there is a wide range of tests that can be performed on serum, some tests require the use of whole blood or plasma. The type of material stored is determined, in most cases, by the types of tests required. The DoDSR has a mission to engage in medical surveillance and support the prevention and control of diseases relevant to the military. Using avian influenza surveillance and related research as an example, studies could be conducted on military service members who have been deployed to countries that have experienced avian influenza outbreaks to determine if any service members have been exposed. Serum stored in DoDSR could be tested to determine exposure by determining whether any service members had developed an antibody response to avian influenza. This information could then be matched with their medical records to see if they had an influenza-like illness during their deployment. Testing for human influenza subtypes is already being undertaken in a similar manner. If the DoD considers this testing fully sufficient for medical surveillance and disease prevention and control purposes, then serum specimens as currently collected and stored most likely are adequate.

However, should the DoD feel that more in-depth study of factors potentially predisposing or protecting service members from infectious diseases such as influenza, or that other biological and chemical threats are worthy of surveillance, then it might consider the addition of specimens that contain DNA and RNA. Serum and plasma are not good sources of genetic material for either DNA or RNA testing. For example, if the DoDSR stored genetic material, it could be used to help determine whether some people have a genotype that makes them more or less susceptible to infection or is a predictor of more severe illness caused by avian influenza. Knowledge of a service member's susceptibility to avian influenza would be useful in multiple ways. A genetic screening tool could be developed to screen service members before deployment to areas susceptible to avian influenza. Susceptible service members could either receive prophylactic treatment to prevent infection or be reassigned to not include deployment to high-risk areas. The knowledge of genotypes could lead to the development of different vaccines for different people. In all of these cases, access to genetic material would be necessary.

Purifying and then storing DNA from all specimens would be cost-prohibitive. However, collecting and storing buffy coat or whole blood are both options, and allow for the later purification/isolation of DNA and RNA. Buffy coat and plasma can both be obtained from the same tube of blood. In this case, a separate tube of blood would be required to be collected from the person if serum were still required. However, HIV testing is possible on plasma, and the resulting plasma could be stored for follow-on testing, instead of serum. If whole blood is stored, it can be collected and stored in two ways, either in liquid form from venipuncture, or as a blood spot, collected on filter paper. For both buffy coat and whole blood in liquid form, the specimens would need to be stored at −80°C or colder to be useful for a range of testing, including purifying genetic material. According to a review by the UK Biobank Sample Handle and Storage Subgroup, dried blood spots (DBS) offer the most stable storage format for DNA in blood. Studies have also shown that RNA can be isolated and assayed from DBS (Zhang and McCabe, 1992; Uttayamakul et al., 2005; Baumann et al., 2005). DBS are commonly stored on filter paper at −20°C with a desiccant to minimize humidity, although they can be stored at 4°C, as well (Mei et al., 2001).

Strategy 17: Change the storage temperature of the DoDSR.

While the current storage temperature of −30°C is adequate for many analytes, it does not adequately maintain the integrity of all of the analytes available for testing in serum (Rai et al., 2005). Proper specimen storage is critical to maintaining specimen integrity, and to be able to perform a broader range of tests. To be more confident in the results of those tests, the serum specimens should be stored at −80°C or colder. As noted in strategy 16, if other fractions are collected and stored, especially for analysis of DNA and/or RNA, at a minimum, −80°C is required to maintain their integrity. DBS are the exception and can be stored at −20/−30°C with a desiccant without loss of information.

Data

Current Status

DMSS is AFHSC's data hub and the sole data link to the DoDSR. DMSS is also the sole custodian of deployment health forms. DMSS is a strictly unclassified database that draws different types of data from several sources, as described in detail in Chapter Four and summarized below. DMSS draws data from several sources and retains such data permanently. According to AMSA interviewees, some of the original data sources do not retain data permanently. DMSS data are de-identified and made available as the Defense Medical Epidemiology Database (DMED) to users outside of AMSA. DMSS includes data related to demographic and administrative details, HIV testing, pre- and post-deployment health assessments, immunizations, and inpatient and outpatient encounters from garrison settings.

Findings

Data quality and data connections are not optimal. Several interviewees commented on the inaccuracy and hence lack of reliability of military data, with one characterizing the problem as "leviathan." Such problems cascade into all military data systems, including DMSS. Solutions to such problems must be recognized by AFHSC and others, but remediation is beyond the purview of AFHSC alone. Interviewees from AMSA and ASD(HA) commented on data missing from DMSS. At the time of our study, AMSA was slowly completing the data entry from paper records for early specimens in the archive. AMSA was also incorporating more data into DMSS from routine inpatient and outpatient medical encounters, including diagnoses and pharmacy actions. Incorporation of laboratory data is vexed by the lack of standardization of laboratory testing and reporting across the department.

Deployment-related health data are lacking. The lack of deployment-related data from theater settings represents a gap of particular concern in DMSS at present. Data of interest include health data, (e.g., from the DNBI database, timely tri-service medical event reporting), clinical encounters as recorded in the AHLTA-T platform, and detailed location data.

DMSS links to classified data pose problems. While both the accuracy and availability of personnel location data are problematic, high-resolution person-specific location data during active theater operations (through the Defense Theater Accountability System, DTAS) is generally classified for at least several months. According to sources in ASD(HA), only the specific location data fields are actually classified. This may be one obstacle to the availability of unclassified location data and timely broader deployment-related data feeds into DMSS. Data classification may also be an obstacle for connecting mortality surveillance data into DMSS. We understand that the Theater Medical Data Store (TMDS) is an unclassified data system that contains unclassified deployment health surveillance data that could be immediately linked to DMSS.

There are opportunities for additional linkages to other military biological specimen collections. During our interviews we discovered and explored potential linkages into DMSS of specimens collected for other purposes and archived elsewhere within the military (that could, through DMSS, be linked to both data and serum repository specimens for specific service members if/as needed). Examples include NHRC's collection of isolates and original throat swab specimens from its febrile respiratory illness surveillance program, the Armed Forces Institute of Pathology (AFIP)

Mortality Surveillance Division's necropsy specimens, and AFIP's National Pathology Repository specimens. At least one of these sources expressed interest in pursuing the potential linkage of such specimens through DMSS and even their availability to complement serum specimens archived by AFHSC. There are probably other relevant specimen archives elsewhere within the military services not uncovered through the RAND team's document review and interviews. In contrast to the generally perceived desirability of DMSS data links for specimens archived elsewhere, there were somewhat divergent views among interviewees regarding storage in the repository of specimens collected for other purposes, e.g., related to specific studies. For example, some expressed interest in collecting and storing specimens from the military's current Millennium Cohort Study overseen by NHRC (involves 1,500 active-duty members, to be followed over 20 years),[1] from which specimens are not being collected. However, another military scientist noted that as the source of repository specimens widens, the nature of the specimens—and hence the standardization of collection and processing procedures—may be compromised, potentially reducing the comparability of specimens that may be selected for subsequent testing.

Data on behavioral risk factors are not available. One interviewee suggested linking behavioral risk factors that may be of interest to acute and/or chronic diseases. Such data are not available through systems currently feeding into DMSS, although we learned that DoD does collect such data. The Survey of Health-Related Behaviors Among Military Personnel has collected behavioral risk data from active-duty members in several cycles since 1980. The survey was extended in 2005 to include reserve component personnel. However, these data are collected anonymously and as such could not be linked to member-specific records in DMSS. The question is whether survey data could be collected in such a way that data could be linked to individual service member records, or whether selected questions could be added to nonanonymous data collection tools such as pre- and post-deployment health assessment forms.

Access to DMSS is limited. Several interviewees commented that they do not use DMSS. Some were distressed that the identified data they send to DMSS is not accessible to them via DMED (which is de-identified and the only database made accessible outside AMSA/AFHSC). Their workaround has been to directly obtain the broad range of needed data from such sources as the Defense Management Data Center (DMDC) and other channels.

Potential Improvement Strategies

Based on our findings, the key actionable questions related to DMSS data concern lack of connections to certain relevant data sources (especially deployment-related data from theater settings) and data links to other DoD biological specimen archives, the

---

[1] Information on the Millennium Cohort Study accessed online. As of January 24, 2008: www.millenniumcohort.org/endorsements.php

desirability and ability to capture relevant behavioral risk information, potential obstacles associated with classified information, and access by military health users outside AMSA to sufficiently detailed data through DMSS.

- What other data sources should be fed into DMSS?
- Should behavioral risk factor data be captured by DMSS, and if so, how?
- How important are classified data elements, and how can desirable classified data be handled within DMSS?
- Can and should access to DMSS be enhanced?

The following strategies address these questions.

Strategy 18: Link additional relevant data sources into DMSS in a reliable and timely manner.

A first step in this strategy would be establishment of criteria to guide decisions regarding new connections to DMSS. Such criteria should begin with meeting requirements specified throughout relevant military policy, especially deployment health data from theater settings. Other criteria could include potential benefits—e.g., the relevance of specific new data elements to meet the (potentially redefined or prioritized) mission and range of uses of DoDSR and DMSS in support of force health protection—weighed against potential challenges—e.g., data classification, delays in data availability, interoperability of data systems. An alternative to this systematic process is simply to identify desired new data (several examples are mentioned above) and then proceed to determine how to feed such data into DMSS. It will then be important to review a current inventory of all military databases and their data content and wiring diagrams to determine the best sources of needed data.

Strategy 19: Connect other military specimen collections into DMSS.

This strategy first involves a canvassing or inventory of potentially relevant specimen collections currently stored across DoD and then assessing the desirability and feasibility of linking them to DMSS (so that analyses based on these specimens could use the DMSS database) or even making those other specimens available for further testing in conjunction with testing of serum from the same service members. Criteria for such assessments could include size and retrievability of specimens, and the nature and degree of incremental benefit that the new specimens themselves, or at least linkages to DMSS, might provide.

Strategy 20: Capture behavioral risk factor information in DMSS.

The first question is the extent to which such information would add relevant value, weighed against the obstacles in obtaining it. The second question would then be how to do so. Two potential options include changing the longstanding and comprehensive military survey mentioned above from anonymous to nonanonymous status or collection of selected data elements via current nonanonymous tools such as the pre- and post-deployment health and periodic health assessment forms. The first option may not be practical, since the survey's procedures and guarantees of anonymity are well established. Addition of selected questions to current forms is feasible but would take considerable administrative effort, including required approval from Washington Headquarters Services/Directorate for Information Operations and Reports for changing the content of any of these forms. Considerations should include the types of behavioral risk data most relevant to surveillance, epidemiological investigation, clinical support, and military health research, the volume of current and projected demand for such data, and the likelihood that information would be truthfully reported (e.g., may be an issue for reporting alcohol or drug use but perhaps less an issue for tobacco use, diet, or physical activity). An appropriately constituted military body should consider the questions related to behavioral risk factor data in greater detail and weigh potential benefits against administrative and other drawbacks before recommending for or against new data collection that might subsequently be linked into DMSS.

Strategy 21: Overcome obstacles to inclusion of classified data elements.

If all relevant data can be obtained from the Theater Medical Data Store, that would be the easiest solution to overcome current limitations ascribed to housing of such data exclusively within classified systems. However, if data are indeed needed from classified systems, there are at least three possible approaches to implementation of this strategy. First, the entire DMSS database could reside and operate within the classified environment and be accessible by others via the SIPRNET. This would require new policy/doctrine and new secure communication facilities, at least for the central AMSA database. The advantages would be access to a broader range of data, most specifically timely, detailed, and person-specific location data during deployments. However, all current DMSS data—and the overwhelming majority of any future DMSS data—are currently unclassified. Permanent residence and operation of DMSS within the classified environment may limit the number of otherwise relevant military users.

A second approach to implementation is a modular one, in which the main DMSS database is maintained within the current unclassified environment but is mirrored into the classified system and linked to classified data elements, on either an as-needed or systematic basis, to permit analyses involving protected data fields. This is particularly relevant to deployment health: to track health in a timely way during ongoing deployments. DMSS is already required to house such information, but currently does not. To fully meet this requirement, AFHSC will require a secure communications facility. Similar arrangements would be needed if the full DMSS database were available outside of AFHSC. It is important for the broader range of DMSS data—including classified data—to be available to relevant users when needed, and for AFHSC to retain oversight of the DMSS database. It is also important to maintain routine operations and access within the unclassified environment. Thus, unclassified and classified versions of DMSS, both maintained by AFHSC, will likely optimize the number and range of military users.

A third option would be to maintain a strictly unclassified DMSS system that incorporates personnel location information once it becomes declassified. Although this is a logistically simpler approach toward the goal of capturing this information, the disadvantages are the delays until sensitive theater information is declassified and made available to unclassified data systems such as DMSS. Such delays would jeopardize time-sensitive clinical management and epidemiological investigation needs.

Strategy 22: Expand access to DMSS.

Expanding access to DMSS beyond AMSA/AFHSC staff can be accomplished in different ways. AMSA already hosted "affiliated analysts" who performed targeted analyses of special interest, e.g., mental health (WRAIR) and deployment health (Deployment Health Support Directorate, under Force Health Protection and Readiness within OSD). If DMSS is made available to remote users, privacy protections must be extended beyond the current central DMSS site to any other sites where DMSS resides or is accessed. This is not a critical factor for the more readily available online DMED database, which includes aggregated and de-identified data.

A first option would be to expand the number of service liaisons and "affiliated analysts" working out of the AFHSC facility and directly accessing DMSS. This would enhance tri-service visibility and operations while also broadening the AFHSC-based staff using the central DMSS database to perform a broad range of relevant analyses needed by individual services as well as DoD-wide. A second option would be to mirror the DMSS database into each service's surveillance hub (or other designated site), with appropriate privacy protections and procedures as specified and followed by AFHSC itself. This would permit direct access by a single site from each service's own location. A third, and related, option would be to broaden DMSS access even further, similar to the range of access now available online for DMED, by web-enabling the data and query systems and controlling its use via password protections. A last approach, and the main one that was in practice through the period of this study, is for all analyses requiring identifiable data to be performed by AMSA staff upon request. Because several interviewees expressed concerns about their access to DMSS itself, this last option is probably the least desirable because it puts the greatest pressure on the small AMSA/AFHSC staff, resulting in less timely and/or a less robust range of analyses from DMSS, and does not fully satisfy external users who prefer to undertake their own analyses.

Users and Uses

Current Status

AMSA and a small number of liaison and periodic "affiliated analyst" staff working out of the AMSA/AFHSC offices were the sole users of the central DMSS database, which has data with individual identifiers (mostly for linking to specimens and for clinical and other support). AMSA converted DMSS into a de-identified database—DMED—for other users. DMED provides aggregated data, mostly from outpatient and inpatient databases. The full range of users of DMSS and DMED has included AMSA (internal research, e.g., seroepidemiology), military researchers (Uniformed Services University of the Health Sciences, WRAIR, U.S. Army Medical Research Institute for Infectious Diseases, Walter Reed Army Medical Center), clinicians (DMSS data only, for individual patient management), the Military Vaccine Agency, Armed Forces Epidemiology Board (now Defense Health Board), and health surveillance hubs (AFIOH, NHRC, GEIS). Serum specimens are available for use by military researchers. Civilian researchers must partner with military counterparts to access the specimen repository. In addition, patients can request their specimens for medical purposes, but the request must come through their physician. If it is a civilian physician, the request needs to go through a military physician to gain access to the specimen and informed consent must be obtained from the patient.

DMSS data and DoDSR specimens have been used for surveillance, outbreak investigation, clinical management, and military research. Typically, single specimens are requested, e.g., for clinical support or to compare with specimens from ongoing investigations. Longitudinal specimens are much less frequently requested. Moreover, requests for AMSA analyses from DMSS data far exceeded the number of requests for serum specimens. Over 120 serum studies were approved by AMSA through early February 2008, mostly for research (and mostly including civilian researchers) and occasionally from policymaking components such as the Defense Health Board and the offices of the service Surgeons General.

Findings

The repository is a "national treasure" that is seriously underutilized and whose value has not yet been fully realized. Data from AMSA indicate that it received approximately 120 requests for specimens between 2001 and January 2008, or an average of about 25 requests per year. Considering the size of the repository (over 43 million specimens) and the valuable linkage to the DMSS database, one can make a strong case that the repository could be used more robustly even if strictly for surveillance and epidemiologic investigation purposes, e.g., systematic comparisons of pre- and post-deployment specimens, cross-sectional or longitudinal surveillance studies for pathogens of interest such as influenza and other respiratory viruses, or epidemiologic investigation of disease outbreaks. Moreover, serum specimens can also theoretically support research studies relevant to military populations, particularly those that aim to assess biological risk factors for post-deployment problems. Interestingly, several interviewees (outside AMSA) had personally used the serum repository for research studies or investigations, including studies on chronic diseases. All of them reported good experiences and high value of the repository. However, these same users felt that the repository was not being used to its full potential.

Underutilization of DoDSR could derive from several potential causes. Since interviewees commented specifically on the underutilization of the DoDSR, we asked them to suggest possible reasons for this. Some commented that military health personnel, especially clinicians, are largely unaware of the repository. Countering this, others expressed concern about managing or accommodating a greatly increased demand. Utilization of the repository may also be due in part to a perceived mismatch between range of missions for DoDSR as defined in policy (and perceived areas of value as expressed by interviewees) and the surveillance mission of AMSA/AFHSC, which oversees DoDSR. For example, some interviewees commented that the serum repository has no role in surveillance or situational awareness, based on a perception of surveillance within a real-time time frame. In contrast, AMSA staff specifically described comparison of pre- and post-deployment specimens as a surveillance function.

The repository is not widely perceived as valuable for (real-time) deployment health, and systematic testing of pre- and post-deployment specimens is not carried out. Since neither DMSS nor DoDSR currently captures real-time data or specimens from deployment settings, they cannot support real-time surveillance. Thus, the main deployment surveillance uses of the DoDSR are comparisons of pre- and post-deployment specimens, e.g., routinely or ad hoc for antibodies to selected infectious disease agents. However, infectious diseases, for which the serum specimens are most relevant, are not proving to be a major health problem in current theater operations. Even chronic disease research studies most often have examined infectious disease markers (antibodies) from serum specimens, looking at potential infectious disease precursors to selected chronic diseases.

Outbreak investigations and research are widely viewed as valuable uses for specimens from the DoDSR. Indeed, one military group commented that the repository is not very valuable because DoD's main focus is operational support, whereas the repository is well suited to support research to improve force health protection, which may not be viewed as operational support, thus limiting—either by perception or in reality—the use of the DoDSR for research. Indeed, several interviewees commented on the great value—and largely untapped potential—of the longitudinal specimens available through the repository. Finally, there were differing views regarding the utility of the repository for clinical support.

The nature and degree of access to DoDSR specimens for civilian research remains an issue. More than one interviewee raised the possibility of making repository specimens more readily available to civilian researchers, including more active use by the Veterans Health Administration. However, others expressed potential concerns with broadening access—other than potentially to the VA—e.g., because of the limited number of aliquots per specimen, risk of deviating from military mission or interests, and complications introduced if any funding for additional repository support (in exchange for increased repository access) might come from nonmilitary sources as a result of opening access beyond the military.

Potential Improvement Strategies

Based on our findings, the key questions related to use of the repository and DMSS data concern underutilization of specimens, for a variety of potential reasons including lack of awareness, lack of consensus regarding appropriate uses of serum specimens (which may be associated in part with the mismatch between the surveillance mission and limited staff size of AMSA/AFHSC versus potential research uses), and lack of value or use in support of deployment health. Another key question concerns the underutilization of multiple/longitudinal serial specimens from the repository.

- Should efforts be made to raise awareness of the repository, especially among military health personnel and similarly among civilian researchers?
- How can the repository be more useful to deployment health?
- How can the longitudinal nature of the serum specimens be used to greatest advantage?

The following strategies address these questions.

Strategy 23: Raise awareness of DoDSR and DMSS.

Information campaigns to raise awareness of DoDSR and DMSS can broaden the user base and increase the use of these resources. Communications efforts can selectively target groups relevant to specific uses, e.g., clinicians for clinical support uses; alternatively, they can take a broader approach to educate the entire military health community and others on the availability and full range of uses of these specimen and data resources. Once the mission and full range of appropriate uses of the repository and DMSS database are prioritized and clarified, information about the availability of and procedures for accessing these resources can be widely disseminated. AFHSC can take the lead for such efforts, including renewed encouragement to its service surveillance hub counterparts to enhance their use of the repository and DMSS resources. Other appropriate entities can also help raise awareness, e.g., the Joint Preventive Medicine Policy Group (for surveillance, investigation, and research uses), TRICARE Management Activity, the offices of the service Surgeons General, and the VA (for clinical support uses), the Uniformed Services University of the Health Sciences and potentially others (for research uses), and/or relevant officials within the Office of the Secretary of Defense such as the Assistant Secretary of Defense for Health Affairs or the Under

Secretary of Defense for Personnel and Readiness. The Deployment Health Centers—NHRC (research) and Walter Reed Army Medical Center (clinical) can also contribute to raising awareness across a broader range of relevant military users. The advantages of this strategy include more robust use of what has been widely acknowledged as a valuable but underutilized military resource. However, increased demand for specimens may lead to more rapid drawdown of available serum aliquots and further burden AFHSC staff. Such disadvantages could be mitigated by other improvement strategies, such as release of smaller aliquots and more robust staffing of AFHSC, including military staff from other services, if/as required to meet an expanded mission or level of demand.

Strategy 24: Coordinate actions to increase the utility of the repository and DMSS for deployment health.

Because military policy (e.g., DoDD 6490.03, DoDD 6490.02E, USD(P&R) Memorandum of April 2003, MCM-0006-02 JCS Memorandum of February 2002) emphasizes the importance of deployment health and requires timely submission of data to DMSS and specimens to the repository, enhancing the use and perceived value of these resources in support of deployment health should be a particular priority, especially the acquisition of relevant data from deployed settings. Based on our analyses and comments from interviewees, implementation of this strategy could involve a number of potential specific actions:

- Fully implement current requirements for timely feeds of relevant deployment health data into DMSS, e.g., DNBI, tri-service medical event reports, data from medical encounters as recorded on DD Form 2766 and via the AHLTA-T platform, and person-specific location information (declassified, with a 60+ day delay, or more timely classified location data requiring a classified version of DMSS, as described in Strategies 18 and 21 above).
- Reinforce communications to the other Deployment Health Centers and to other relevant users (including the VA) regarding the availability and utility of the DoDSR and DMSS in support of deployment health—especially if relevant new data are fed into DMSS and on a more timely basis.
- Increase the systematic analysis and reporting on trends specifically linked to deployments, especially based on the new data linkages from theater environments as noted above. A more resource-intensive strategy would be proactive and systematic testing of pre- and post-deployment serum specimens (all or a relevant specimen) for infectious disease surveillance purposes. This could be done by AMSA, other service surveillance hubs, other Deployment Health Centers, the VA, or other relevant military health personnel.

Strategy 25: Broaden civilian access to the specimen repository, including VA and other researchers.

There are both incremental and broad approaches to implementing this strategy. For example, a first priority might be to raise awareness and use of DMSS and/or the repository among the VA medical/health community, either selectively, e.g., for clinical support to individuals, or more broadly, e.g., for the full range of uses of the data or serum specimens: individual medical management, public health investigation, or research for health or clinical management policy for service members on active duty or separated. This incremental approach maintains the strong military focus of the specimen and data resources, while extending access beyond the DoD itself. While AFHSC provides deployment health form data to the VA for separating service members, more of the VA health community, including its leadership, should be made aware of its access to DMSS and DoDSR resources.

A broader approach to this strategy would be to make the data and/or specimen resources more available to civilian researchers, either passively (make aware but do not actively advertise) or actively (advertise availability). Further, civilian researchers could still be required to partner with a military co-principal investigator or not, and the proposed research could be required to demonstrate relevance to the military or not. Combinations of these various options could result in narrow to broad expansion of non-DoD users of DMSS data and/or specimens. However, human subjects protection becomes an increasing issue and challenge if/as use expands beyond surveillance and investigation purposes and beyond military users. Purely civilian research not directly tied to military priorities may prove to be an obstacle for ethical reasons, unless human subjects protection issues can be resolved. (Strategy 6 proposes ways to address human subject protections.) Military leadership may wish to consider this issue more comprehensively by asking an appropriately constituted group to review the different options and their associated implications and offer more specific policy recommendations.

Strategy 26: Increase use of serial specimens from the repository.

Since serial specimens (beyond strictly paired specimens) are of greatest value for longitudinal analysis, and because both the DoDSR and DMSS are longitudinal in nature, these resources provide unique opportunities for surveillance and research drawing upon a longitudinal population sampling design. Assuming the continued legitimacy of research use for the specimens, the awareness-raising efforts described in Strategy 23 would be appropriate. Military health leadership and appropriately constituted groups could help raise awareness across the military and VA health/medical research and surveillance communities, with a particular focus on the unique large and serial nature of the serum repository. The Uniformed Services University of the Health Sciences could also play a key role in both promoting and using specimens for appropriate longitudinal studies.

Chapter Highlights

The DoDSR and DMSS have already demonstrated their value to military health surveillance and to military health more broadly. Nonetheless, this systematic review has led to the identification of potential ways to further improve the use and hence value of these resources. Figure 6.3 presents a summary of the improvement strategies described in this chapter.

Several of the improvement strategies described above are interdependent, so they should not be considered purely independently. Based on the review in this chapter alone, a "package" of improvement strategies could include the following:

- Explicit clarification of the mission and authorized uses of the DoDSR and DMSS to include the relative priority for surveillance, clinical support, investigation, and research in support of force health protection, deployment health, and the health of separated service members.
- Communications to promote a common understanding of the meaning of such terms as "surveillance" and "research" as they relate to the DoDSR and DMSS in particular, and to promote use of these resources.
- More timely availability of specimens from DoDSR.

Figure 6.3
Summary of Potential Improvements in DoDSR/DMSS System Elements and Characteristics

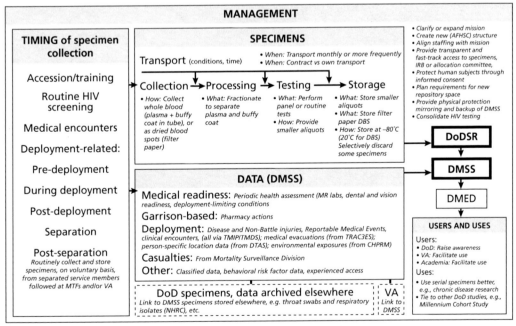

- Establishment of clear criteria and procedures for accessing DoDSR specimens.
- Linkages of new data sources to DMSS, particularly health and other data from ongoing deployments.
- Expanded access to DMSS.
- Ongoing collection of specimens, on a voluntary basis, from separated service members followed at MTFs or through the VA health system.
- Archiving of new blood-derived specimens that reliably retain genetic material for future testing, including biomarkers and tests yet to be identified and developed.
- Final determination of location, space, and other requirements for the new repository.

The discussion and recommendations in the following chapter aim to consolidate and suggest priorities for consideration by military authorities.

CHAPTER SEVEN

Synthesis and Recommendations

It is clear from document review and interviews with a broad range of staff throughout DoD that AMSA was a good steward of the DoDSR and DMSS resources and used them well in support of military medical surveillance in particular. However, the goal of this study was to help identify opportunities to make even better use of these resources in addressing military health needs now and into the future.

Our analyses have uncovered specific opportunities to better fulfill current requirements, especially to close gaps in the content and efficiency of medical surveillance. The largest gap relates to data from deployed settings, which figures prominently within the strategies described in the previous chapter and the recommendations presented here. Our report also describes the larger context for DoD surveillance, which is important to consider as potential improvements in the DoDSR and DMSS components are contemplated, i.e., medical surveillance together with occupational and environmental health surveillance constituting "health surveillance," and these all within the even larger context of "comprehensive health surveillance," which encompasses the entire career of service across all locations. Beyond surveillance, we have also identified specific ways to position the DoDSR and DMSS resources to better serve the military of the future: planning now for changes that will permit a wider range of uses to improve not only surveillance but also clinical management and research in support of force health protection. Taken as a whole, the recommendations we offer below suggest that the DoDSR and DMSS could benefit from improved oversight and management to ensure that they function within the strategic goals of the Military Health System, and have access to the needed data systems as well as other resources needed on an ongoing basis. This chapter draws from the preceding chapter and packages our findings and proposed strategies for improvement into six main recommendations, which are again organized based on our conceptual framework. Decisions at the level of both the Under Secretary of Defense and AFHSC will cascade across the recommendations we offer here, affecting the direction of the decisions as well as the magnitude of change.

Management

1. Clarify and communicate the missions of DoDSR and DMSS both within and beyond DoD.

There is a mismatch between congressional direction for the use of the DoDSR and the DMSS data system as articulated in several enactments of the National Defense Authorization Act and the articulation of the mission and use of the DoDSR and DMSS by AMSA. Clear articulation by AFHSC and a common understanding across DoDSR and DMSS users of the full range of uses for these resources and their relative priority—including surveillance, epidemiologic investigation, clinical management, and research related to both infectious and noncommunicable diseases—should lead to their more efficient and robust use within DoD. Further, the mission of DoDSR and DMSS to collect specimens and data could also extend beyond DoD active or reserve populations to include continuation of data and specimen collection on a voluntary basis from service members followed in Military Treatment Facilities and/or the Veterans Health Administration system. To harness the full potential of the DoDSR and DMSS resources, AFHSC should establish the relative priority for the different uses and users of these resources and then make these explicit by communicating widely across DoD and into related research and epidemiologic communities if/as appropriate.

2. Empower, structure, and resource the organizational oversight of DoDSR and DMSS so that they can fulfill the full range of missions.

In Chapter Two we describe how DoD's own policy envisioned a tri-service surveillance center, and we believe the vision and guidance to be relevant and timely today. Specifically, a 1999 ASD(HA) memorandum described the migration of DMSS toward a "DoD Medical Surveillance Agency" collecting all theater medical surveillance and treatment data collected by the services, unified and specified commands, and individual commands within the services. Further, DMSS was directed to provide access to personnel and health surveillance data to other agencies involved in medical surveillance and health research (ASD(HA), September 30, 1999).

As we describe in the Authors' Note to our report, DoD officially established the AFHSC in late February 2008. We learned from our interviews that the intent for this organization is to encompass DoD-wide medical surveillance activities within one organization, by combining AMSA, GEIS, and the Deployment Health Support Directorate of OSD(HA). Review of the AFHSC Concept of Operations indicated that the new organization will also encompass the broader range of health surveillance components and activities, i.e., including occupational and environmental health in garrison and deployment settings (although details of these were largely beyond the focus of this study). The organization is envisioned to be a tri-service surveillance agency, although we understand that there were concerns among the services about how to staff such an agency and what the appropriate oversight of the agency should be.

We hope that the AFHSC will be able to connect the various experts, contracts, and systems that are required not only for its primary surveillance mission but also for the full range of uses (primarily within the military by also extending into the civilian community) for the DoDSR and DMSS resources it manages through its executive agency function, including surveillance, epidemiologic investigation, clinical management, and research. Further, we hope that the chain of command and oversight for this organization will be such that it can receive guidance and resources from policymakers responsible for all of these functions, e.g., the ASD(HA), Surgeons General, and Army Medical Research and Materiel Command, in order to ensure proper alignment with current Military Health System strategy and resources and medical research and service health priorities as relevant to DoDSR and DMSS. The AFHSC should be configured and staffed to provide the support needed by all users, and especially those within DoD, supporting execution of the designated missions for DoDSR and DMSS. In Chapter Six we described approaches to leveraging new staff resources if needed.

Data

3. Create an integrative data plan for comprehensive health surveillance.

Ideally, AFHSC should develop a construct wherein all the various data required for medical surveillance and broader health surveillance would be linked and would reflect the underlying tenets of comprehensive health surveillance. Currently, as we describe in Chapter Three, there are many data systems within the services and COCOMs that are being used for various medical and other health surveillance functions. There are issues related to data classification and connections that impede DMSS from being a fully functional deployment medical surveillance tool, although the capabilities that are not resident in DMSS are being conducted at other sites and with other systems. However, there seems to be no overarching and comprehensive data plan prescribing integration of all relevant heath surveillance data. Such a plan should address issues such as connectivity to occupational and environmental health surveillance systems, both within the garrison and deployed settings, increasing data collection along a service member's period of service and beyond, and fully realizing policy efforts to facilitate access to surveillance and other data by the VA.

Regarding DMSS specifically, over the past several years AMSA effectively increased the number of data feeds into DMSS and expanded the breadth of its surveillance reporting accordingly. However, several relevant datasets remain unconnected to DMSS, thus limiting the full execution of AFHSC's surveillance mission and limiting DoD's ability more broadly to take advantage of the full range of value offered by DMSS. The highest priorities for new data linkages into DMSS relate to deployment health, serving primarily but not exclusively a deployment health surveillance mission. These data sources include theater-based reportable medical events, clinical encounters (via AHLTA-T), and disease and non-battle injury (DNBI) data, all available via the Theater Medical Information Program (TMIP). We understand that relevant health surveillance data can possibly be made available to DMSS via the unclassified Theater Medical Data Store; however, this was not confirmed during the period of our study. Member-specific deployment location information is also important and available through the Deployment Theater Accountability System, though the data in this system are classified. For data that cannot be made available via these systems, options for linking classified data into DMSS include time-delayed incorporation of declassified location data or near-real-time incorporation of classified data. The latter imposes potentially new requirements on AFHSC, i.e., for a secure communications facility to house either the original or a mirrored version of the DMSS database. Other relevant linkages to consider are to existing DoD biological specimen archives such as isolates and original nasal swab specimens maintained by NHRC from its Febrile Respiratory Illness Surveillance system and pathology and necropsy specimens maintained by the Armed Forces Institute of Pathology in the National Pathology Repository. Consideration should also be given to collecting and archiving specimens from the recently initiated Millennium Cohort Study, overseen by NHRC. More robust linkages in both directions between DMSS and the VA health system should also be considered, to the extent that the missions of DoDSR and DMSS are expanded beyond strictly active duty and reserve populations. Also, consideration should be given to whether and how behavioral risk factor data should be collected and fed into DMSS, as discussed in Chapters Four and Six. Finally, as technology develops new ways of testing for the presence and use of chemical or biological weapons, DMSS might be tailored to contribute to surveillance or research for these potential threats. Because there are many current data sources that might be tapped for deployment health surveillance, and there may be more in the future, the new AFHSC would be better positioned to fully execute its mission if it were included in the Military Health System information requirements process currently managed at the TRICARE Management Activity.

Better protection of DMSS's physical infrastructure and the integrity of the data (i.e., to resist physical or cyber threats to the DMSS database) is also needed. We recommend that strong consideration be given not only to assuring adequate housing of the data system, but also to systematic and frequent offsite backup and even parallel mirroring of the DMSS database, to assure its integrity in response to any threat that may arise, as occurred in late January 2008.

Specimens

4. Enhance the utility of specimens.

The DoDSR serum specimens continue to serve well their original purpose of HIV serosurveillance. However, as we discussed in Chapter Two, as early as 1997, the

DoD made a decision to continue to use serum to meet new requirements related to biological specimens for deployment health surveillance. The sera permit examination of deployment-related exposures to and investigations of infectious agents; they are not particularly useful for time-sensitive environmental exposures for which biomarkers are only fleetingly present. And, as military health research becomes broader and more technologically sophisticated, the limitations of current serum specimens become more apparent: researchers increasingly recognize the importance of genetic material for current and future research into a range of acute and chronic conditions. Serum specimens as presently stored in the DoDSR at −30°C do not reliably preserve genetic material. Therefore, it is timely at this juncture, as the current repository lease expires and the new AFHSC looks toward serving the longer-term needs of the Military Health System, to consider ways to enhance the utility of the DoDSR specimens.

There may be some incremental value in storing future serum specimens at −80°C (note that storage of current specimens at colder temperatures would not change the availability of analytes for future testing). Even greater value would be derived from whole blood specimens, e.g., stored in liquid form or as dried blood spots, or storage of buffy coat fractions in which the quantity of genetic material is substantially greater (see description in Chapter Five). Storage requirements for dried blood spots are modest and incrementally the easiest. Alternatively, archiving of plasma and buffy coat could be accomplished through collection of blood specimens in a tube that allows fractionation into plasma and buffy coat; plasma can be used in place of serum for routine HIV testing and for essentially all other tests currently performed on DoDSR serum specimens. Storage of both plasma and buffy coat at −80°C reflects current best industry practices for preservation of genetic material and other relevant blood-derived analytes. However, adoption of this alternative would mean costly new repository requirements for future specimens, i.e., walk-in freezers would not be possible for storage at −80°C. Nonetheless, the near-term expiration of the current repository lease and potential relocation provides a timely opportunity for military leadership to think carefully about the needs of the Military Health System into the future and determine whether new kinds of specimens should be archived, to better serve a broader range of mission areas for this valuable military resource.

5. Plan for the next repository facility.

Depending on decisions related to the strategies described in Chapter Six and the other recommendations here, DoD should begin now to define the requirements for the next repository, following expiration of the current lease in 2010. Factors to take into consideration include the time horizon for the next repository (e.g., 20 years or more), the annual rate of specimen acquisition (which would increase if specimens are to be collected from members following separation), the types of specimen to be archived (e.g., serum or plasma, buffy coat, whole blood in liquid form or as dried blood spots), and desired storage temperature (e.g., $-30°C$ or $-80°C$). All of these influence the size and configuration of the future repository and hence the requirements for future repository space.

Users and Uses

6. Raise awareness of and expand access to DoDSR and DMSS.

The use of DoDSR and DMSS resources to date is perceived to be limited, and a key reason offered by military interviewees is that awareness of these resources across DoD is limited. For example, one military medical officer noted that military clinicians are largely unaware of these resources in support of clinical management. Likewise, a senior health official within the VA system was largely unaware of the rich specimen and data resources available through DoDSR and DMSS. Several interviewees suggested broad or targeted "educational campaigns" to raise awareness and use of these resources.

Access to specimens is also perceived to have been limited because of what some considered a lack of fully transparent criteria for release of specimens. A remedy for this could include development and dissemination of updated and transparent criteria and procedures for accessing DoDSR specimens and DMSS data. The cost associated with obtaining specimens from the repository, $20 per specimen, has also been cited as a barrier for civilians wanting to tap into the DoDSR for the purposes of research.

In terms of expanding use, the first priority should probably be for military health users within DoD, followed by more robust use by the VA. DoD should carefully consider whether and how to expand use to civilian researchers, while protecting individual privacy, the overall military health mission, and availability of remaining specimens as more users draw down the number of aliquots from a given specimen. Finally, efforts should be made to take better advantage of the longitudinal nature of the DoDSR inventory, e.g., through clarifying the legitimate use of DoDSR for research and sensitizing military health researchers to the availability of these serial specimens and linked data.

Conclusions

The goal of this study was to help identify opportunities to make even better use of DoDSR and DMSS resources in addressing military health needs now and into the future. Our analyses uncovered specific opportunities to better fulfill current requirements, especially to close gaps in the content and efficiency of medical surveillance. The largest gap relates to data from deployed settings, which figures prominently within the strategies we describe in the report and our recommendations. Beyond surveillance, we have also identified specific ways to position the DoDSR and DMSS resources to better serve the military of the future: planning now for changes that will permit a wider range of uses to improve not only surveillance but also clinical management and research in support of force health protection. Taken as a whole, our recommendations suggest that the DoDSR and DMSS could benefit from improved oversight and management to ensure that they function within the strategic goals of the Military Health System, and have access to the needed data systems as well as other resources they need to fulfill their mission. Creation of the new AFHSC (after this study was completed) seems to be a good step in that direction, though detailed study of any new directions AFHSC may be taking are beyond the scope of the present study. There are key decisions that need to be made at the Under Secretary of Defense level which will cascade across the recommendations we offer here, affecting the direction of the decisions as well as the magnitude of change.

AMSA was a responsible custodian for the DoDSR and DMSS, characterized by multiple interviewees as "national treasures" whose full potential has yet to be fully harnessed. Creation of the new AFHSC and relocation of the repository offer the opportunity to consider how the DoDSR and DMSS resources can be used to even greater advantage to support military health now and into the future. This study took a systematic approach to analysis of current characteristics and opportunities for improvement. Some of our recommendations are relatively easy to implement, while others are more ambitious. Nonetheless, we feel that implementation of all of these recommendations will allow the AFHSC to better fulfill its current requirements, serve a broader range of legitimate mission areas, and position the DoDSR and DMSS resources for valuable service well into the future.

Summary of Legislation and Policy Establishing Requirements for DoDSR and DMSS

Source and Date	Key Provisions
ASD(HA) Memorandum (December 5, 1985) (Superseded by DoDD 6485.1, March 19, 1991.)	*The DoD HTLV-III Testing Program*
DoDD 6485.1 (Originally issued March 19, 1991, reissued August 10, 1992.) (Superseded by DoDI 6485.01, October 17, 2006. Not included here.)	*Human Immunodeficiency Virus-1 (HIV-1)* • Establishes DoD's HIV program • Does not mention serum repository
DoDI 6490.3 (August 7, 1997) (Superseded by DoDI 6490.03, August 11, 2006. See below.)	*Implementation and Application of Joint Medical Surveillance for Deployments* • Mandates joint comprehensive medical surveillance for active service, including reserve component, before/during/after deployments • Medical surveillance includes Armed Forces Serum Repository and data • CHPPM charged with operation of repository and data system • Specifies use of specimens exclusively in relation to military operations • Charters establishment of Joint Preventive Medicine Policy Group
DoDD 6490.2 (August 30, 1997) (Superseded by DoDD 6490.02E, October 21, 2004. See below.)	*Joint Medical Surveillance* • Designates Army as executive agent for deployment medical surveillance and serum repository • Requires that medical and personnel data systems be compatible with military medical surveillance • Charges CHPPM to perform periodic (not routine) epidemiologic studies of data derived from the serum repository
Public Law 105-85 (November 18, 1997)	*National Defense Authorization Act, FY98* • Requires DoD to draw blood specimens pre- and post-deployment and maintain a central archive of health records relating to deployments

Source and Date	Key Provisions
ASD(HA) Memorandum (October 6, 1998)	*Policy for Pre- and Post-Deployment Health Assessments and Blood Samples* • Establishes the pre- and post-deployment health assessment for all military members, including collection of blood specimens
Public Law 105-261 (October 17, 1998)	*National Defense Authorization Act, FY99* • Authorizes establishment of a center for deployment health • Requires the center to collect and study data in order to determine the effect of deployment on health
ASD(HA) Memorandum (November 6, 1998)	*Tri-Service Reportable Events* • Requires the use of a tri-service reportable events list, established by a joint working group, the Joint Preventive Medicine Policy Group, by all services • Directs reportable events to be integrated into DMSS • Requires DMSS to make data available to all services for further analyses
Joint Chiefs of Staff MCM-251-98 (December 4, 1998)	*Deployment Health Surveillance and Readiness* • Provides standardized procedures for assessing health readiness for deployment • Establishes deployment health surveillance procedures
ASD(HA) Memorandum (February 3, 1999)	*Policy for DoD Global, Laboratory-Based Influenza Surveillance* • Designates DMSS as the influenza surveillance database
ASD(HA) Memorandum (September 30, 1999)	*Establishment of DoD Centers for Deployment Health* • Continues the use of DMSS for medical surveillance • Describes DMSS migration strategy toward "DoD Medical Surveillance Agency" • Requires all theater medical surveillance and treatment data be forwarded to DMSS • Requires remote access to DMSS be provided to NHRC and others involved in surveillance and military health research • Requires TRICARE Management Activity to provide unrestricted access to applicable Military Health System data and support DMSS as appropriate • Defines DMSS as the comprehensive longitudinal, relational, epidemiology database for the study of deployment health • Establishes Deployment Health Working Group
ASD(HA) Memorandum (October 25, 2001)	*Updated Policy for Pre- and Post-Deployment Health Assessments and Blood Samples* • Updates original HA Policy 99-002 (October 1998) to apply all deployment-related health assessments and specimen collections for all reserve component personnel called to active duty for ≥30 days • Stipulates use of DD Forms 2795 and 2796 across all services

Source and Date	Key Provisions
Joint Chiefs of Staff MCM-0006-002 (February 1, 2002) (Supersedes MCM-251-98, December 4, 1998. See above.)	*Updated Procedures for Deployment Health Surveillance and Readiness* • Justifies comprehensive health surveillance within force health protection • Requires all deployment health surveillance data be sent to DMSS • Notes the value of near-real-time DNBI data • Alludes to DD Form 2766 (also as deployed medical record) • Requires commanders provide DNBI and reportable medical events data and post-deployment health assessment forms on a timely basis • Requires DNBI data be sent weekly and simultaneously to COCOM Surgeon and to service surveillance centers and DMSS
USD(P&R) Memorandum (April 22, 2003) (Canceled by DoDI 6490.03, Deployment Health, August 11, 2006. See below.)	*Enhanced Post-Deployment Health Assessments* • Requires face-to-face post-deployment health assessment, using revised DD Form 2796 • Shortens the interval for post-deployment health forms and serum specimens to 30 days following redeployment home
ASD(HA) Memorandum (May 1, 2003)	*Tracking Post-Deployment Health Assessments* • Requires services to put in place weekly reporting of completion rates of post-deployment health assessments
ASD(HA) Memorandum (January 9, 2004)	*Policy for DoD Deployment Health Quality Assurance Program* • Requires AMSA to send at least monthly reports to OSD/Deployment Health Support Directorate on deployment health assessment data • Establishes baseline metrics relating to deployment health assessment forms and post-deployment sera • Requires services to establish deployment health QA programs
ASD(HA) Memorandum (May 21, 2004)	*Automation of Pre- and Post-Deployment Health Assessment Forms* • Requires plans for electronic submission of DD Forms 2795 and 2796 and integration into an eventual Military Health System Central Data Repository
DoDD 6200.04 (October 9, 2004. Certified current as of April 23, 2007.)	*Force Health Protection (FHP)* • Requires "routine annual health, medical, and dental assessments," "annual assessment of IMR," (para 4.3.1.3) pre- and post-deployment and separation health assessments • Specifies DoD maintain a central repository for biospecimens to be used in clinical care, forensics, and epidemiologic studies • Specifies that DoD "pursue scientific and technological advancements to improve and protect the health of the force through medical research, development, clinical investigations, technology insertion, and appropriate acquisition strategies" (para 4.5)

Source and Date	Key Provisions
DoDD 6490.02E (October 21, 2004. Certified current as of April 23, 2007.) (Supersedes DoDD 6490.2, August 30, 1997. See above.)	*Comprehensive Health Surveillance (CHS)* • Specifies surveillance across service members' careers, duty locations, and spectrum of health risks, interventions and outcomes • Defines comprehensive, health, medical and occupational and environmental surveillance • Specifies CHS as important to FHP • Requires medical and personnel data systems be designed to be compatible with military health surveillance objectives • Requires surveillance data be transferred to VA upon separation • Broadens scope of DoDSR beyond deployment surveillance • Calls (again) for establishment of Joint Preventive Medicine Policy Group • Reiterates Army as executive agent for DoDSR, DMSS
Public Law 108-375 (October 28, 2004)	*National Defense Authorization Act, FY05* • Reduces time frame for collection of pre-deployment specimens from 12 months to 120 days prior to deployment, as an interim standard to be re-examined by DoD • Requires DoD to maintain a theater health record • Requires DoD to evaluate its deployment medical tracking and health surveillance systems, which included a scientific review of the utility of blood sampling procedures for exposure detection • Requires DoD to prescribe policy relating to classification of in-theater data
DASD(FHP&R) Memorandum (January 27, 2005)	*Requirements for Blood Samples Before and After Deployments* • Responds to the NDAA FY05 • Requires compliance with interim blood sampling time frames of no more than 120 days pre-deployment and 30 days post-deployment • Describes request to AFEB and CDC to answer questions posed by Congress in NDAA FY05
ASD(HA) Memorandum (March 10, 2005)	*Post-Deployment Health Reassessment* • Requires post-deployment reassessment 3–6 months following return to home station (new DD Form 2900) • Requires automated form be submitted to AMSA for DMSS • Defines purpose as proactive identification of health concerns emerging over time following deployments, especially mental health

Source and Date	Key Provisions
AFEB 2005-03 (April 28, 2005)	*Response to Questions Pertaining to the Utility of the Requirements to Collect and Store Pre- and Post-Deployment Serum Specimens* • Recommends serum with WBC as an "acceptable and cost effective specimen for the analysis of most biological and some chemical agents of current and future interest to [DoD]" (para 7) • Recommends widespread awareness and use of DoDSR • Recommends consideration of an "oversight panel to help govern access to the archived specimens" (p. 3, question 2) • Supports current pre- and post-deployment windows for specimen collection and continuation of 100% sampling for these
DoDI 6025.19 (January 3, 2006)	*Individual Medical Readiness* • Establishes a baseline of six elements describing individual medical readiness across all services and applicable to all service members • Requires ASD(HA) to oversee tri-service IMR program and to report data
ASD(HA) Memorandum (March 14, 2006) (Rescinds DASD(FHP&R) Memorandum, January 27, 2005. See above.)	*Policy for Pre- and Post-Deployment Serum* • Reestablishes timing of pre-deployment serum specimen collection up to one year prior to deployment, and post-deployment collection within 30 days after deployment
DoDI 6490.03 (August 11, 2006) (Supersedes DoDI 6490.3, August 7, 1997. See above.)	*Deployment Health* • Reiterates requirements for post-deployment and separation serum specimens and forwarding deployment health assessment forms to DMSS • Requires COCOM commanders to provide timely reporting of DNBI and other medical information (Note: reporting destination not specified) • Requires DoDSR/DMSS to make "individual and Service aggregated data" available to military services (5.8.11) • Specifies that DMSS provide periodic trend analysis reports and integrated Reportable Medical Events data to service components • Requires that all deployment-phase medical encounters be recorded on DD Form 2766 or equivalent • Requires daily review of DNBI data and tri-service reportable medical events reported to COCOM or service component "via currently approved and available electronic data collection and transmission devices" (E4.A2.4) • Requires, to the extent feasible, that deployment health data "be collected and maintained in DoD-approved automated health information management systems" (E4.A2.4) (Note: No system specified)

Source and Date	Key Provisions
DoDD 6490.02E (October 21, 2004. Certified current as of April 23, 2007.) (Supersedes DoDD 6490.2, August 30, 1997. See above.)	*Comprehensive Health Surveillance (CHS)* • Specifies surveillance across service members' careers, duty locations, and spectrum of health risks, interventions and outcomes • Defines comprehensive, health, medical, and occupational and environmental surveillance • Specifies CHS as important to FHP • Requires medical and personnel data systems be designed to be compatible with military health surveillance objectives • Requires surveillance data be transferred to VA upon separation • Broadens scope of DoDSR beyond deployment surveillance • Calls for establishment of Joint Preventive Medicine Policy Group • Reiterates Army as executive agent for DoDSR, DMSS
Joint Chiefs of Staff MCM 0028-07 (November 2, 2007)	*Updated Procedures for Deployment Health Surveillance and Readiness* • Focuses particularly on occupational/ environmental surveillance and risk assessment • Specifies that disease and injury data be reported on timely basis and electronically where feasible (through Patient Encounter Modules [PEMs] that feed into JMeWS, AHLTA-T or JPTA) • Mentions "Armed Forces Health Surveillance Center" as one of several "upstream authorities," and separately notes USACHPPM, AFIOH, and NEHC as service surveillance hubs • Does not explicitly specify DMSS as destination for any deployment health data

Published Research Conducted from Sera at the DoD Serum Repository or Based on Data Drawn from the DMSS, as of January 2008

1. Nevin RL, Shuping EE, Frick KD, Gaydos JC, Gaydos CA. Cost and effectiveness of chlamydia screening among male military recruits: Markov modeling of complications averted through notification of prior female partners. *Sex Transm Dis.* 2008 (in press).

2. Nevin RL, Carbonell I, Thurmond V. Device-specific rates of needlestick injury at a large military teaching hospital. *Am J Infect Control.* 2008 (in press).

3. Bloom MS, Hu Z, Gaydos JC, Brundage JF, Tobler SK. Differences in outpatient pelvic inflammatory disease rates between Army and Navy recruits. *Am J Prev Med.* 2008 Jun (in press).

4. Nevin RL, Pietrusiak PP, Caci JB. Prevalence of contraindications to mefloquine use among USA military personnel deployed to Afghanistan. *Malaria Journal.* 2008; 7:30 (Epub February 11, 2008, at http://www.malariajournal.com/content/7/1/30).

5. Niebuhr DW, Millikan AM, Cowan DN, Yolken R, Li Y, Weber NS. Selected infectious agents and risk of schizophrenia among U.S. military personnel. *Am J Psych.* 2008; 165:99–106.

6. Niebuhr DW, Millikan AM, Yolken R, Li Y, Weber NS. Results from a hypothesis generating case-control study: herpes family viruses and schizophrenia among military personnel. *Schizophrenia Bulletin.* 2007 Dec 21; (Epub ahead of print).

7. Eick AA, Hu Z, Wang Z, Nevin RL. Incidence of mumps and immunity to measles, mumps and rubella among U.S. military recruits, 2000–2004. *Vaccine.* 2007 Dec 4; (Epub ahead of print).

8. Hsu LL, Nevin RL, Tobler SK, Rubertone MV. Trends in overweight and obesity among 18-year-old applicants to the United States Military, 1993–2006. *J Adolesc Health* 2007 Dec; 41(6):610–2.

9. Milliken CS, Auchterlonie JL, Hoge CW. Longitudinal assessment of mental health problems among active and reserve component soldiers returning from the Iraq War. *JAMA.* 2007; 298(18):2141–8.

10. Brundage JF, Shanks GD. What really happened during the 1918 influenza pandemic? The importance of bacterial secondary infections. (correspondence). *J Infect Dis.* 2007 Dec 1; 196:1717–8.

11. Cook MB, Zhang Y, Graubard BI, Rubertone MV, Erickson RL, McGlynn KA. Risk of testicular germ-cell tumours in relation to childhood physical activity. *Br J Cancer.* 2007 Nov 20; (Epub ahead of print).

12. Majka DS, Deane KD, Parrish LA, Lazar AA, Barón AE, Walker CW, Rubertone MV, Gilliland WR, Norris JM, Holers VM. The duration of pre-clinical rheumatoid arthritis-related autoantibody positivity increases in subjects with older age at time of disease diagnosis. *Ann Rheum Dis.* 2007 Nov 1; (Epub ahead of print).

13. Eckart RE, Shry EA, Atwood JE, Brundage JF, Lay JC, Bateson TF, Grabenstein JD. Smallpox vaccination and ischemic coronary events in healthy adults. *Vaccine.* 2007 Oct 17; (Epub ahead of print).

14. Nevin RL, Niebuhr DW. Rising hepatitis A immunity in U.S. military recruits. *Mil Med.* 2007 Jul; 172(7):787–93.

15. Ciminera P, Brundage JF. Malaria in U.S. military forces: a description of deployment exposures from 2003 through 2005. *Am J Trop Med Hyg.* 2007 Feb; 76(2):275–9.

16. McGlynn KA, Sakoda LC, Rubertone MV, Sesterhenn IA, Lyu C, Graubard BI, Erickson RL. Body size, dairy consumption, puberty, and risk of testicular germ cell tumors. *Am J Epidemiol.* 2007 Feb 15; 165(4):355–63.

17. Purdue MP, Sakoda LC, Graubard BI, Welch R, Chanock SJ, Sesterhenn IA, Rubertone MV, Erickson RL, McGlynn KA. A case-control investigation of immune function gene polymorphisms and risk of testicular germ cell tumors. *Cancer Epidemiol Biomarkers Prev.* 2007 Jan; 16(1):77–83.

18. Munger KL, Levin LI, Hollis BW, Howard NS, Ascherio A. Serum 25-hydroxyvitamin D levels and risk of multiple sclerosis. *JAMA.* 2006 Dec 20; 296(23):2832–8.

19. Brundage JF, Johnson KE, Lange JL, Rubertone MV. Comparing the population health impacts of medical conditions using routinely collected health care utilization data: nature and sources of variability. *Mil Med.* 2006 Oct; 171(10):937–42.

20. McGlynn KA, Zhang Y, Sakoda LC, Rubertone MV, Erickson RL, Graubard BI. Maternal smoking and testicular germ cell tumors. *Cancer Epidemiol Biomarkers Prev.* 2006 Oct; 15(10):1820–4.

21. Arcari CM, Nelson KE, Netski DM, Nieto FJ, Gaydos CA. No association between hepatitis C virus seropositivity and acute myocardial infarction. *Clin Infect Dis.* 2006 Sep 15; 43(6):e53–6. Epub 2006 Aug 8.

22. Brundage JF. Cases and deaths during influenza pandemics in the United States. *Am J Prev Med.* 2006 Sep; 31(3):252–6.

23. Hoge CW, Auchterlonie JL, Milliken CS. (In reply to letters to the editor). Mental health after deployment to Iraq or Afghanistan. *JAMA.* 2006 Aug 2; 296(5):516.

24. Brundage JF. Interactions between influenza and bacterial respiratory pathogens: implications for pandemic preparedness. *Lancet Inf Dis.* 2006 May; 6(5):303–12.

25. Isenbarger DW, Atwood JE, Scott PT, Bateson T, Coyle LC, Gillespie DL, Pearse LA, Villines TC, Cassimatis DC, Finelli LN, Taylor AJ, Grabenstein JD. Venous thromboembolism among United States soldiers deployed to southwest Asia. *Thromb Res.* 2006; 117(4):379–83.

26. Hoge CW, Auchterlonie JL, Milliken CS. Mental health and occupational impact of deployments to Iraq and Afghanistan: findings from population-based post-deployment screening and surveillance. *JAMA.* 2006 Mar 1; 295(9):1023–32.

27. Pablo K, Rooks P, Nevin R. Benefits of serologic screening for hepatitis B immunity in military recruits. (Correspondence) (Letter to the Editor). *J Infect Dis.* 2005 Dec 15; 192(12):2180–1.

28. Scott PT, Niebuhr DW, McGready JB, Gaydos JC. Hepatitis B immunity in United States military recruits. *J Infect Dis.* 2005 Jun 1; 191(11):1835–41.

29. Levin LI, Munger KL, Rubertone MV, Peck CA, Lennette ET, Spiegelman D, Ascherio A. Temporal relationship between elevation of epstein-barr virus antibody titers and initial onset of neurological symptoms in multiple sclerosis. *JAMA.* 2005 May 25; 293(20):2496–500.

30. Ascherio A, Rubertone M, Spiegelman D, Levin L, Munger K, Peck C, Lennette E. Notice of retraction: "Multiple sclerosis and Epstein-Barr virus" (JAMA 2003; 289:1533–6). *JAMA*. 2005 May 25; 293(20):2466.

31. Arcari CM, Gaydos CA, Nieto FJ, Krauss M, Nelson KE. Association between Chlamydia pneumoniae and acute myocardial infarction in young men in the United States military: the importance of timing of exposure measurement. *Clin Infect Dis*. 2005 Apr 15; 40(8):1123–30. Epub 2005 Mar 14.

32. Acinetobacter baumannii infections among patients at military medical facilities treating injured U.S. service members, 2002–2004. *MMWR*. 2004 Nov; 19:53(45):1063–67.

33. Arness MK, Eckart RE, Love SS, Atwood JE, Wells TS, Engler RJ, Collins LC, Ludwig SL, Riddle JR, Grabenstein JD, Tornberg DN, for the Department of Defense Smallpox Vaccination Clinical Evaluation Team. Myopericarditis following smallpox vaccination. *Am J Epidemiol*. 2004 Oct 1; 160(7):642–51.

34. Munger KL, DeLorenze GN, Levin LI, Rubertone MV, Vogelman JH, Peck CA, Peeling RW, Orentreich N, Ascherio A. A prospective study of Chlamydia pneumoniae infection and risk of MS in two cohorts. *Neurology*. 2004; 62:1799–1803.

35. McClain MT, Arbuckle MR, Heinlen LD, Dennis GJ, Roebuck J, Rubertone MV, Harley JB, James JA. The prevalence, onset, and clinical significance of antiphospholipid antibodies prior to diagnosis of systemic lupus erythematosus. *Arthritis Rheum*. 2004 Apr; 50(4):1226–32.

36. Arbuckle MR, James JA, Dennis GJ, Rubertone MV, McClain MT, Kim XR, Harley JB. Rapid clinical progression to diagnosis among African-American men with systemic lupus erythematosus. *Lupus*. 2003; 12(2):99–106.

37. Lange JL, Campbell KE, Brundage JF. Respiratory illnesses in relation to military assignments in the Mojave Desert: retrospective surveillance over a ten-year period. *Mil Med*. 2003; 168:1039–43.

38. Arbuckle MR, McClain MT, Rubertone MV, Scofield RH, Dennis GJ, James JA, Harley JB. Development of autoantibodies before the clinical onset of systemic lupus erythematosus. *New Eng J Med*. 2003 Oct 16; 349:1526–33.

39. Severe acute pneumonitis among deployed U.S. military personnel—Southwest Asia, March–August 2003. *MMWR*. 2003 Sep; 12:52(36):857–9.

40. Hoge CW, Brundage JF, Engel CC Jr, Messer SC, Orman DT. Reply to letter to the editor. *Am J Psychiatry*. 2003 Jun 1; 160(6):1191–2.

41. Halsell JS, Riddle JR, Atwood JE, Gardner P, Shope R, Poland GA, Gray GC, Ostroff S, Eckart RE, Hospenthal DR, Gibson RL, Grabenstein JD, Arness MK, Tornberg DN, and the Department of Defense Smallpox Vaccination Clinical Evaluation Team. Myopericarditis following smallpox vaccination among US military personnel. *JAMA*. 2003 Jun 25; 289(24):3283–9.

42. Lange J, Lesikar S, Rubertone MV, Brundage JF. Comprehensive systematic surveillance for adverse effects of Anthrax Vaccine Adsorbed, 1998–2000. *Vaccine*. 2003; 21(15):1620–8.

43. Levin LI, Munger KL, Rubertone MV, Peck CA, Lennette ET, Spiegelman D, Ascherio A. Multiple sclerosis and Epstein-Barr virus. *JAMA*. 2003; 289:1533–6.

44. Wasserman GM, Grabenstein JD, Pittman PR, Rubertone MV, Gibbs PP, Wang LZ, Golder LG. Analysis of adverse events after anthrax immunization in US Army medical personnel. *J Occup Environ Med*. 2003 Mar; 45(3):222–33.

45. Silverberg MJ, Brundage JF, Rubertone MV. Timing and completeness of routine testing for antibodies to human immunodeficiency virus, type 1, among active duty members of the U.S. Armed Forces. *Mil Med*. 2003 Feb; 168(2):160–4.

46. Wilson ALG, Lange JL, Brundage JF, Frommelt RA. Risk factors for accidental death among male soldiers. *Prev Med*. 2003 Jan; 36:124–30.

47. Brundage JF, Ryan MAK, Feighner BH, Erdtmann FJ. Meningococcal disease among U.S. military servicemembers in relation to routine uses of vaccines with different serogroup-specific components, 1964–1998. *Clin Infect Dis*. 2002 Dec 1; 35(11):1376–81.

48. Rubertone MV, Brundage JF. The Defense Medical Surveillance System and the Department of Defense Serum Repository: glimpses of the future of comprehensive public health surveillance. *Am J Pub Hlth*. 2002 Dec; 92(12):1900–4.

49. Silverberg M, Frommelt A, Lange J, Brundage J, Rubertone M, Winterton BS. Lightning-associated injuries and deaths—United States Armed Forces, 1998–2001. *MMWR*. 2002 Sep 27; 51(38):859–62.

50. Hoge CW, Lesikar SE, Guevara R, Lange J, Brundage J, Engel CC, Messer SC, Orman DT. Mental disorder diagnoses among U.S. military personnel in the 1990s: association with high health care utilization and early military attrition. *Am J Psychiatry*. 2002 Sep; 159(9):1576–83.

51. Campbell KE, Brundage JF. Effects of climate, latitude, and season on the incidence of Bell's palsy, US Armed Forces, October 1997–September 1999. *Am J Epidemiol*. 2002 Jul 1; 158(1):32–9.

52. Brundage JF, Kohlhase KF, Gambel JM. Hospitalization experiences of U.S. servicemembers before, during, and after participation in peacekeeping operations in Bosnia-Herzegovina. *Am J Ind Med.* 2002 Apr; 41(4):279–84.

53. Sanchez JL, Binn LN, Innis BL, Reynolds RD, Lee T, Mitchell-Raymundo F, Craig SC, Marquez JP, Shepherd GA, Polyak CS, Conolly J, Kohlhase KF. Epidemic of adenovirus-induced respiratory illness among US military recruits: epidemiologic and immunologic risk factors in healthy, young adults. *J Med Virol.* 2001 Dec; 65(4):710–8.

54. Barker TL, Richards AL, Laksono E, Sanchez JL, Feighner BH, McBride WZ, Rubertone MV, Hyams KC. Serosurvey of Borrelia burgdorferi infection among U.S. military personnel: a low risk of infection. *Am J Trop Med Hyg.* 2001 Dec; 65(6):804–9.

55. Paris RM, Bedno SA, Krauss MR, Keep LW, Rubertone MV. Weighing in on type 2 diabetes in the military: characteristics of U.S. military personnel at entry who develop type 2 diabetes. *Diabetes Care.* 2001 Nov; 24(11):1894–8.

56. Andreotti G, Lange JL, Brundage JF. The nature, incidence, and impact of eye injuries among US military personnel: implications for prevention. *Arch Ophthalmol.* 2001 Nov; 119(11):1693–7.

57. Arbuckle MR, James JA, Kohlhase KF, Rubertone MV, Dennis GJ, Harley JB. Development of anti-dsDNA autoantibodies prior to clinical diagnosis of systemic lupus erythematosus. *Scand J Immunol.* 2001 Jul-Aug; 54(1-2):211–9.

58. Sanchez JL Jr, Craig SC, Kohlhase K, Polyak C, Ludwig SL, Rumm PD. Health assessment of U.S. military personnel deployed to Bosnia-Herzegovina for Operation Joint Endeavor. *Mil Med.* 2001 Jun; 166(6):470–4.

59. Hyams KC, Riddle J, Rubertone M, Trump D, Alter MJ, Cruess DF, Han X, Nainam OV, Seeff LB, Mazzuchi JF, Bailey S. Prevalence and incidence of hepatitis C virus infection in the US military: a seroepidemiologic survey of 21,000 troops. *Am J Epidemiol.* 2001 Apr 15; 153(8):764–70.

60. Barnett SD, Brundage JF. Incidence of recurrent diagnoses of Chlamydia trachomatis genital infections among male and female soldiers of the US Army. *Sex Transm Infect.* 2001 Feb; 77(1):33–6.

61. Preston DM, Levin LI, Jacobson DJ, Jacobsen SJ, Rubertone M, Holmes E, Murphy GP, Moul JW. Prostate-specific antigen levels in young white and black men 20 to 45 years old. *Urology.* 2000 Nov 1; 56(5):812–6.

62. Brundage JF, Kohlhase KF, Rubertone MV. Hospitalizations for all causes of U.S. military service members in relation to participation in Operations Joint Endeavor and Joint Guard, Bosnia-Herzegovina, January 1995 to December 1997. *Mil Med.* 2000 Jul; 165(7):505–11.

63. Jones BH, Perrotta DM, Canham-Chervak ML, Nee MA, Brundage JF. Injuries in the military: a review and commentary focused on prevention. *Am J Prev Med (suppl).* 2000 Apr; 18(3S):71–84.

64. Arness MK, Feighner BH, Canham ML, Taylor DN, Monroe SS, Cieslak TJ, Hoedebecke EL, Polyak CS, Cuthie JC, Fankhauser RL, Humphrey CD, Barker TL, Jenkins CD, Skillman DR. Norwalk-like viral gastroenteritis outbreak in U.S. Army trainees. *Emerg Infect Dis.* 2000 Mar–Apr; 6(2):204–7.

65. Craig SC, Pittman PR, Lewis TE, Rossi CA, Henchal EA, Kuschner RA, Martinez C, Kohlhase KF, Cuthie JC, Welch GE, Sanchez JL. An accelerated schedule for tick-borne encephalitis vaccine: the American Military experience in Bosnia. *Am J Trop Med Hyg.* 1999 Dec; 61(6):874–8.

66. Barraza EM, Ludwig SL, Gaydos JC, Brundage JF. Re-emergence of adenovirus type 4 acute respiratory disease in military trainees: report of an outbreak during a lapse in vaccination. *J Infect Dis.* 1999 Jun; 179(6):1531–3.

67. Ludwig SL, Brundage JF, Kelley PW, Nang R, Towle C, Schnurr DP, Crawford-Miksza L, Gaydos J. Prevalence of antibodies to adenovirus, serotypes 4 and 7, among unimmunized US Army trainees: results of a retrospective nationwide seroprevalence survey. *J Infect Dis.* 1998 Dec; 178(6):1776–8.

68. Brundage JF. Military preventive medicine and medical surveillance in the post-cold war era. *Mil Med.* 1998 May; 163(5):272–7.

69. Brundage JF, Gunzenhauser JD, Longfield JN, Rubertone MV, Ludwig SL, Rubin FA, Kaplan EL. Epidemiology and control of acute respiratory diseases with emphasis on group A beta-hemolytic streptococcus: a decade of U.S. Army experience. *Pediatrics.* 1996 Jun; 97(6 Pt 2):964–70.

Key Characteristics of Six Biological Specimen Repositories

National Health and Nutrition Examination Survey (NHANES)

Mission

The Centers for Disease Control and Prevention's (CDC) National Center for Health Statistics (NCHS) conducts the National Health and Nutrition Examination Survey (NHANES). NHANES began in 1959 after the National Health Survey Act of 1956 (NHANES, 2008) established a continuing health survey of the people of the United States. The mission continues to be to collect information about the health and diet of the American people, including population-based information on diseases and associated risk factors, e.g., nutritional, behavioral, environmental, genetic (CDC NCHS, 2008). It provides an in-depth survey and assessment of the health status of Americans through personal interviews, standardized physical exams, and laboratory tests. NHANES is the only nationally representative health survey with linked biological specimens in the United States.

Collection

Currently, the NHANES surveys collect information over the course of two years on a nationally representative sample (approximately 5,000–7,000 participants per year). Initially NHANES was a periodic survey, but as of 1999, NHANES has become a continuous annual survey. NHANES collects specimens annually but only releases data files every two years (mostly due to disclosure and reliability issues), thus the data release cycle for the continuous studies is described as NHANES 1999–2000, NHANES 2001–2002, etc. Though the survey content can change every two years, the laboratory methods are held as constant as possible across cycles to be consistent with the data release cycles, and to provide the potential for combination of two or more two-year cycles for greater statistical reliability (CDC NCHS, 2008).

Individuals are recruited from various counties and geographic locations. A mobile examination center (MEC), which includes a laboratory, travels to each location throughout the two-year survey period to interview participants, conduct a physical examination, and collect the specimens. Currently, NHANES collects blood, urine, and other specimen types (such as vaginal swabs from consenting females) from each participant. Between three to eleven blood collection tubes (number and size/type of tubes differ by age) are collected from each individual and are processed in the MEC into serum, plasma, and whole blood aliquots. Whole blood specimens for DNA purification are collected from consenting adults age 20 or older.

Storage and Processing

Some of the vials are stored at 4°C depending on the intended laboratory test, while most serum/plasma vials are stored at –20°C or –30°C until shipment to CDC or a contract laboratory. Most specimens are shipped once a week. There are currently 23 contract or CDC laboratories that conduct a variety of laboratory tests. In the current cycle, three to fifteen vials of serum (0.5–1.0mL aliquots) and plasma (0.5mL aliquots) per survey participant are sent to the CDC and ASTDR (the Agency for Toxic Substances and Disease Registry) Specimen Packing Inventory and Repository (CASPIR) in Lawrenceville, Georgia, for long-term storage in liquid nitrogen (–196°C). CASPIR has approximately 5 million specimens in storage, of which approximately 550,000 are from NHANES. Specimens that have been sent from laboratory testing during the survey are returned to a Fisher BioService Repository (located in the Washington, D.C., metro area) operated under NCHS contract. These specimens have gone through at least two freeze-thaw cycles and are subsequently stored at –80°C. Researchers who submit proposals for use of the NHANES specimens are requested to utilize these specimens, if possible. Those who need pristine, never-thawed specimens must justify the use of these specimens that are stored at CASPIR.

Testing

NHANES conducts a standard set of approximately 550 laboratory tests on different blood fractions and other biological specimens. These tests include standard clinical assessments such as biochemical, hematology, and immunology based tests. Results from the tests are provided to the participant in a hard copy report of findings; other laboratory tests are for research purposes and include a variety of public health topics (such as environmental health). During the second phase of NHANES III (1991–1994), NHANES 1999–2002, and NHANES 2007 to present, the laboratory protocols have included the collection of DNA specimens. The NHANES III specimens (cell lysates from Epstein-Barr transformed cell lines) are stored in liquid nitrogen at CASPIR. Purified DNA specimen aliquots from NHANES 1999–2002 and 2007 onward are stored at –80°C at the National Center for Environmental Health Molecular Biology laboratory, which is the processing laboratory for NHANES DNA specimens. These specimens are being used for genetic research proposals, with proposals accepted twice a year.[1]

---

[1]   Tests vary by the age and gender of participant. For general tests, see www.cdc.gov/nchs/about/major/nhanes/testcomp.htm.

Use of Specimens

Starting in 1999, all participants must complete a separate informed consent form allowing for the use of their specimens in future research. Separate consent for genetic research is obtained from individuals age 20 and older. All proposals for use of the NHANES specimens must undergo a technical review and a CDC Ethics Review Board review. Proposals for DNA specimens must also be reviewed by a Secondary Review Panel which performs a programmatic review. NHANES usually approves 5–8 nongenetic proposals a year from CDC, other federal agencies, and nonfederal investigators, with approximately 5,000–10,000 specimens distributed with each proposal.

Laboratory test results are publicly released at the end of the two-year data collection cycle with the questionnaire and examination data; unless the results are determined to be a disclosure risk (i.e., sexually transmitted infection test results for adolescents are considered a disclosure risk). Results that are considered a disclosure risk can be accessed in the NCHS Research Data Center. Results from the stored specimen are also released publicly on the NCHS/NHANES web site. Genetic test results can only be accessed in the NCHS Research Data Center.[2]

The NHANES results are usually available one year after a two-year data collection cycle. There is a nominal fee to investigators of $2 per serum/plasma/urine specimen sent by the repository. For an NHANES III DNA specimen the cost is approximately $6, and for an NHANES 1999–2002 specimen it is $8. The fee recoups some of the costs associated with the collection and storage of the specimen, and collection and processing of the accompanying data.

United Kingdom Biobank

Mission

UK Biobank is a repository funded both by government (United Kingdom Department of Health and National Health Service) and by private charities (Wellcome Trust, British Heart Foundation, and Cancer Research UK) (UK Biobank, 2008). The concept of the Biobank was initially discussed in 1999, with feasibility studies completed in 2001. The Biobank is a research initiative with the goals of improving the prevention, diagnosis, and treatment of a wide range of serious life-threatening chronic illnesses, such as cancer, heart diseases, diabetes, arthritis, and forms of dementia. The UK Biobank is intended to be used as a prospective epidemiological resource, in part to support a variety of different types of studies, including nested control studies, case control studies, etc. The UK Biobank posts its main protocol online, and many of the details presented here are available in this protocol (UK Biobank, 2008).

---

[2]   A list of currently available NHANES III single nucleotide polymorphisms for secondary data analysis can be obtained from http://www.cdc.gov/nchs/nhanes/genetics/genetic.htm.

Collection

In April 2007, the UK Biobank began the main phase of recruitment, collecting data and biological specimens from a large sample of people in the UK. The goal is to recruit up to 500,000 people between the ages of 40–69 from all over the UK. The UK Biobank identifies individuals through the UK National Health Service Records; once an "assessment center" is set up, UK Biobank invites all appropriate individuals living within a 10-mile radius to participate. Over the initial course of the study (2007–2010), 35 centers will be set up, with six centers being open at any given time and each center being open for six months. Participants are reimbursed for any travel costs. Personnel at the clinics complete an informed consent process with potential participants, and then conduct a health questionnaire and collect physical measurements and biological specimens from each participant in a process that takes approximately 90 minutes. There are also provisions that allow researchers to ask for and obtain additional specimens from particular participants in the future, depending on research objectives.

Processing

The study collects blood and urine from each participant. Six different bar-coded vacutainer tubes of blood and one container of urine are collected. At the assessment center, prior to shipping, one tube of blood is centrifuged to separate plasma, and one tube is centrifuged to separate serum. All of the tubes are sent daily, via overnight courier, to a centralized processing center. Five of the blood specimen tubes and the urine tube are stored and transported at 4°C until further processing on the next day. Temperature integrity is maintained by a sensor that records temperature every ten minutes, while the specimen is in transit. One blood specimen tube is collected in acid citrate dextrose and transported at 18°C. At the central processing center, each tube is processed and then immediately tested or stored. Hematology tests are run on one tube, since those tests cannot be completed on stored specimens. The rest of the tubes are separated into specific fractions (plasma, buffy coat, RBC, serum, whole blood), split into 1.4ml aliquots, and stored at either –80°C or in liquid nitrogen, usually a 60/40 split, respectively. The tube collected in acid citrate dextrose is processed with a cryoprotectant and stored in liquid nitrogen with the intention of potentially purifying the lymphocytes and converting them into immortal cell lines.[3]

Storage

The Biobank repository is a "two-archive" system. The first archive is the "working archive" and can hold up to nine million specimens at –80°C, and has an automated, robotic retrieval system. The automated retrieval system operates such that specimens are never exposed to temperatures above –20°C until after retrieval. In addition, the

---

[3]   Immortalized cell lines offer the greatest opportunity to harvest large amounts of genetic material for research studies.

robotic retrieval system helps with accurate storage and retrieval of specimens. The system includes a computerized inventory, and when the robotic system retrieves a specimen, it checks that specimen against the bar-code and verifies it as the correct specimen. The second archive is the "storage archive," which stores specimens in liquid nitrogen (–196°C) and has a storage capacity of six million tubes. These specimens are manually retrieved.

One of the goals of the UK Biobank is to facilitate genetic research, including studying the relationship between genes and the environment (UK Biobank, 2004). As a result, the working group that developed guidelines for specimen collection and storage considered many different sources of genetic material. The buffy coat fraction containing WBC is the primary fraction being stored for genetic testing. The blood stored in cryprotectant in liquid nitrogen offers a potential to study very large quantities of genetic material by making the cells immortal, thereby giving researchers an unlimited supply of genetic material for research. However, that process is expensive and will only be performed on specific specimens of interest.

Use of Specimens

Researchers from academic, commercial, charity, and public-sector organizations, both nationally and internationally, can request access to specimens stored at the Biobank. Currently, UK Biobank scientific protocols and operational procedures, as well as proposed uses of the repository specimens, are reviewed by an appropriate ethics committee, e.g., Central Office of Research, National Health Service Research Ethics Committee ("UK Biobank Ethics and Governance Framework," 2007). As a part of the access policy, researchers will be charged a nominal fee for specimens. During the 2006 fiscal year (during which UK Biobank conducted pilot studies), UK Biobank had a total operating cost of £4,038,748 (approximately $8 million as of the writing of this report) of which £22,041 (approximately $43,000 as of the writing of this report) was governance costs. The operating cost covered some of the development costs and the pilot studies (recruitment, collection, testing, and storage of specimens).

National Heart, Lung, and Blood Institute (NHLBI)

Mission

The National Institutes of Health's National Heart, Lung, and Blood Institute (NHLBI) supports programs in basic research, clinical investigations, and trials related to diseases of the heart, lung, blood vessels, blood, and sleep disorders. Within NHLBI, the Division of Blood Diseases and Resources manages the NHLBI Biologic Specimen Repository (Biorepository). The NHLBI Biorepository acts as a central repository for specimens collected by NHLBI studies that are performed around the country by various research institutions. The purpose of the NHLBI Biorepository is to facilitate research in the areas of heart, lung, and blood. The mission of the Biorepository is to acquire, store, and distribute biological specimens to the scientific community using standardized processes and procedures described in the NHLBI Biorepository Operational Guidelines. There are approximately four million plasma, serum, cellular, or tissue specimens. Eighty percent of the specimens are from blood transfusion safety programs,[4] and the remaining 20 percent are from various other NHLBI cardiovascular and pulmonary programs; individual study inventories range from 4,500 to 2.5 million specimens (NHLBI Factbook, 2006). In 2006, $1,031,572 was allocated to the NHLBI Biorepository contractor for repository operations (NHLBI Factbook, 2006). More background information on the repository and the various studies can be found on the NHLBI web site (see the Bibliography).

Collection and Storage

Because the NHLBI Biorepository contains specimens from a variety of different clinical studies, the material type, collection, processing, testing, longitudinal parameters, and storage of specimens is varied. Study collections contain different combinations of material types (whole blood, plasma, serum, WBC, platelets, RBC, bronchoalveolar lavage, urine, and tissue). Specimens are stored in mechanical freezers at −80°C, in the vapor phase of liquid nitrogen (−135°C to −190°C), or at room temperature depending on the material type and storage medium. In addition, the specimens might be linked to a variety of health information, including clinical and laboratory test result parameters.

For a study collection to be housed in the NHLBI Biorepository, informed consent must be received from all the study participants with specimens in the collection. NHLBI supplies individual studies with language for their informed consent documents to help the studies develop appropriate language for storing of specimens for future research in a repository. In addition, NHLBI provides assistance to research investigators on the information that should be included in an informed consent document regarding the storage and future use of specimens by the scientific community. NHLBI also reviews study documents on describing specimen collection, aliquots, storage, shipping, and tracking to help investigators build study collections that will be of use to the general scientific community.

Use of Specimens

Access to data and specimens at NHLBI depends on which of two study periods a given collection occurs in. The proprietary period lasts until NHLBI receives the study data following a posted limited-access data policy (NHLBI Limited Access Dataset, 2008).

---

[4] NHLBI's Division of the Blood Diseases and Resources, Transfusion Medicine and Cellular Therapeutic Branch has supported various prospective and retrospective studies on blood donors and recipients since the 1970s in an effort to keep the U.S. blood supply safe for transfusions.

The open period follows the proprietary (limited access) period—the duration varies by study type. During the proprietary period, outside investigators can gain access to a study only by collaborating with the study investigators. During the open period, the specimens are available to all qualified investigators in the wider scientific community. NHLBI staff initially screen all applications to ensure that the proposals are complete and have the required IRB approval from their home institutions. The NHLBI Biorepository Allocation Committee reviews all requests for specimens during the open period, while the parent study (usually the Steering Committee) reviews requests for specimens during the proprietary period. The Allocation Committee includes a chair and co-chair with experience in biorepository, the laboratory, and epidemiological methodologies, an ethicist, two ad hoc members who have expertise in the specific research area under review, and one investigator from the original study that collected the specimens. The committee is a virtual committee, which does not meet in person, and the ad hoc and original study investigator can change for each new request, or set of requests, for a given study. From 1999 to 2004, a total of 67,715 specimens were distributed to various investigators.

Division of Retrovirology at Walter Reed Army Institute of Research

Mission
WRAIR conducts research intended to support the U.S. Army and DoD to improve biomedical knowledge and technologies. The main mission of the Retrovirology Division within WRAIR is the prevention of HIV-1 disease in the active component. As part of this, they study the epidemiology of HIV globally; develop diagnostic and immunologic assays to support vaccine development; are involved in HIV vaccine development and testing; and conduct research on treating and caring for HIV-infected individuals (U.S. Military HIV Research Program, 2008). The U.S. Military HIV Research Program Repository stores specimens from patients who have participated in various HIV clinical trials run through WRAIR.

Collection, Processing, and Storage
Currently the retrovirology laboratory has multiple research sites in Africa, South America, and Asia. These research sites focus on conducting vaccine trials, with most of the participants being local residents. At each site, whole blood is collected from patients and fractionated into plasma, serum, and WBC within six hours of collection. These specimens are processed and stored at −80°C at each research site, after which they are batched and shipped to the United States in liquid nitrogen. Upon arrival they are cataloged and stored in liquid nitrogen in the U.S. Military HIV Research Program Repository. Once specimens arrive at the repository they are aliquoted into 1.8mL cryovial tubes. WBC aliquots are stored in liquid nitrogen, while plasma and

serum aliquots are stored at −80°C. The repository has approximately 1 million specimens, with 310,000 stored in liquid nitrogen and the rest stored at −80°C. The yearly acquisition rate for WBC is between 15,000 and 20,000, and between 30,000 and 60,000 for plasma and serum specimens.

Use of Specimens

The clinical data associated with each specimen are dependent upon the research protocol. However, generally, demographic and HIV status is collected, and further testing parameters dependent on the research hypothesis. For most studies, longitudinal specimens are collected (baseline, prior to vaccine, post vaccine, etc.) and a variety of tests (HIV, other viral tests, etc.) are completed on the specimens depending on the study protocol.

All the participants in the vaccine and other research trials sign an informed consent form, which includes consent to use their specimens in research, and all of the research study protocols undergo an IRB approval process in the host country. The repository does not have a separate IRB to oversee the storage of specimens. If outside collaborators (those not initially included in the original study protocol) want access to data or specimens, they must propose amendments to the study protocol, which would have to undergo an additional IRB review from their home institution and the IRB in the host country, as well as receive consent from the principal investigator. Of the few requests granted, the average number of specimens distributed for a given study ranged from 40 to 300. Records are kept of all requests and transactions.

Armed Forces Institute of Pathology: Department of Defense DNA Registry

Mission

The Armed Forces Institute of Pathology (AFIP) is a tri-service DoD agency specializing in pathology consultation, education, and research as well as a referral center for expert pathology diagnostics for the U.S. Armed Forces (AFIP, 2008). AFIP houses the DoD DNA Registry, which is used for the identification of human remains. The DoD DNA Registry consists of a laboratory (the Armed Forces DNA Identification Laboratory) and a repository (the Armed Forces Repository of Specimen Samples for Identification of Remains). The DoD DNA registry provides scientific consultation, research, and education services in the field of forensic DNA analysis, with the goal of ensuring that "the United States would never again have to entomb the remains of an unknown American" (AFIP DoD DNA Registry, 2008). While the specimens in this repository are not used for research, the repository is included here as another example of a military repository and because of its expertise in the storage and testing of specimens for genetic information.

Collection and Processing

The AFIP DNA repository was established in 1992 and, under DoDD 5154.24, collects and maintains blood specimens suitable for DNA analysis from all active component service members, reserve component service members, U.S. Coast Guard personnel, as well as some DoD civilian employees and DoD contractors who support the military in hostile foreign environments (AFIP DoD DNA Registry, 2008). To date, the repository has collected and stores over 5 million specimens. Blood is collected either via finger prick or venipuncture, and two spots are collected on Whatman filter paper. The specimens are allowed to dry for at least 20 minutes at room temperature prior to packaging in individual shipping pouches with desiccant for shipping. All specimens are supposed to be shipped to AFIP within 10 days of collection.[5] Once they arrive at the repository, specimens are checked for completeness of the personal information provided, to include signature of the donor, to attest to the identity of the donor at collection and acknowledge the reading of the informed consent and privacy act statement. A service member's information is checked against the Defense Enrollment Eligibility Reporting System (DEERS) to determine they are eligible for DoD benefits enrollment prior to the specimen being vacuum sealed in an individual pouch with a desiccant to keep it dry and then stored in a two-story freezer at –20°C (Gillert, 1998). The specimens are assigned a unique accession number that serves as a location identifier within the repository. Currently, a quality assurance plan is being reviewed to determine if specimens can be stored at room temperature without affecting the yield and quality of the DNA on the cards.

Informed consent, in the form of privacy act statement acknowledgement, is obtained prior to specimen collection. On a case-by-case basis, service members can request to not have their DNA stored based on religious reasons. The blood is stored to be used only for remains identification and cannot be used for any other purpose per federal law except in support of a criminal investigation, which requires specific criteria to be met, to include the issuance of a federal court order. In the event of a service member's death, disposition of the card becomes the responsibility of the primary next of kin.

deCODE

Mission

deCODE, a private biopharmaceutical company headquartered in Reykjavik, Iceland, was founded in 1996. The goal of the company is to discover genetic variants associated with increased risk of common diseases, and to apply these discoveries to develop DNA-based tests predicting disease risk, as well as drugs targeting the biological

---

5   For collection instructions, see www.afip.org/Departments/oafme/dna/afrssir/.

pathways that are affected by these genetic variants. The company conducts genome-wide, population-based gene discovery work using the population of Iceland as its primary study cohort. Approximately 60 percent of the adult population of Iceland—or 140,000 people—have taken part in one or more of deCODE's gene discovery studies, which cover more than 50 common diseases. Informed consent is obtained from all participants who are asked to participate in research on specific disease areas, though most also sign an informed consent for their genetic data to be used in cross-disease studies as well. All of deCODE's research protocols are reviewed by the Icelandic medical ethics committee, a government body that serves in the capacity of a national IRB. All data on individuals used in deCODE's research is anonymized by the Icelandic Data Protection Authority (DPA), a government body using an encryption system that generates discrete PIN numbers for individuals in order that genetic, medical, and genealogical data can be correlated while still protecting the privacy of participants as set out under European Union directives.

Collection

Specimens are typically collected from patients with particular illnesses or disease characteristics, as well as from family members with and without the disease in question. deCODE frequently runs encrypted patient lists from Iceland's national health care service against a nationwide genealogical database built by the company (encrypted using the same key) to select patients who would be most informative for genetic analysis. The PINs of these patients are then sent back through the DPA, decrypted, and the names sent to doctors in the health service who contact individuals and ask them if they would be willing to participate in a particular study. Participants go to an offsite, deCODE-sponsored clinic, where, after signing an informed consent form, five vials of blood are collected and a health questionnaire is administered. The health questionnaires are typically focused around the particular disease/study, with a few broad application questions. Physicians who are involved with a given research program customarily also take detailed and standardized clinical data relevant to the condition under study. All biological specimens and medical information is anonymized via the DPA before being sent to deCODE.

Processing and Storage

deCODE currently stores over 500,000 biological specimens from both Icelanders and foreigners taking part in its studies via collaborations with clinicians in many countries. Virtually all of these specimens are in the form of whole blood and/or purified DNA. From each participant, five vials of whole blood are collected. One vial is processed into purified DNA and aliquoted into an average of ten 2mL tubes that are stored at 4°C. There is no time restriction on storage length for the purified DNA, but the general rule of thumb practiced by deCODE is that if an aliquot of purified DNA has been stored for less than a year at 4°C, then it can go directly into the research cohort. If an aliquot has been stored longer than a year, it must go through a quality control test before being included in the research cohort. The four other vials are stored as whole blood in 10mL tubes in their repository, called the Secure Robotized Sample Vault (SRSV), at –25°C. All specimens are bar-coded and encrypted. The SRSV can store tubes in a variety of sizes, in customized racks. A robot pulls specimens from the racks and delivers them through an access port in the side of the SRSV, which helps maintain the specimens at a constant temperature.

deCODE adds anywhere between 12,000 and 60,000 new specimens each year from Icelandic and outside participants. They have created three cross-referencable databases that enable the company to analyze correlations between genetic variations and medical data from participants, in the context of comprehensive nationwide genealogical data assembled from public domain sources. deCODE collects informed consent from all participants. deCODE has longitudinal aspects to its research but this is not standard practice; the company is very research-project dependent. deCODE does not send out specimens to outside researchers or share raw data with other research organizations. deCODE researchers do, however, provide services to outside researchers in genotyping and structural biology, and the company markets certain technologies and know-how it has developed for protecting, analyzing, and storing large quantities of specimens and data.

Bibliography

Armed Forces Epidemiology Board, Memorandum, "Responses to Questions Pertaining to the Utility of the Requirements to Collect and Store Pre- and Post-Deployment Serum Specimens," *AFEB* 2005-03, April 28, 2005.

Armed Forces Institute of Pathology. As of March 4, 2008:
http://www.afip.org

Armed Forces Institute of Pathology, Department of Defense DNA Registry. As of December 2009:
http://www.afip.org/consultation/AFMES/AFDIL/index.html

Army Medical Surveillance Activity/Directorate of Epidemiology and Disease Surveillance/ U.S. Army Center of Health Promotion and Preventive Medicine, "Guidelines for Collecting, Maintaining, Requesting, and Using Specimens Stored in the Department of Defense Serum Repository," May 29, 2003.

Baumann, S., et al., "Standardized Approach to Proteome Profiling of Human Serum Based on Magnetic Bead Separation and Matrix-Assisted Laser Desorption/Ionization Time-of-Flight Mass Spectrometry," *Clin Chem*, Vol. 51, No. 6, June 2005, pp. 973–980.

Centers for Disease Control and Prevention, National Center for Health Statistics, "National Health and Nutrition Examination Survey." As of March 4, 2008:
http://www.cdc.gov/nchs/nhanes.htm

Congressional Budget Office (CBO), "The Health Care System for Veterans: An Interim Report," December 2007, p. 1. As of January 24, 2008:
http://www.cbo.gov/ftpdocs/88xx/doc8892/12-21-VA_Healthcare.pdf

deCODE, "deCODE's Population Approach." As of July 13, 2009:
http://www.decode.com/Population-Approach.php

Department of Defense—Global Emerging Infections Surveillance and Response System, "Annual Report for Fiscal Year 2006."

Department of Defense—Global Emerging Infections Surveillance and Response System, "The DoD Worldwide Influenza Surveillance Program." As of November 12, 2007:
http://www.geis.fhp.osd.mil/GEIS/SurveillanceActivities/Influenza/influenza.asp

Department of Defense Directive (DoDD) 6485.1, "Human Immunodeficiency Virus-1 (HIV-1)," August 10, 1992.

Department of Defense Directive (DoDD) 5124.2, "Under Secretary of Defense for Personnel and Readiness," 1994.

Department of Defense Directive (DoDD) 6490.2, "Joint Medical Surveillance," August 30, 1997.

Department of Defense Directive (DoDD) 3216.02, "Protection of Human Subjects and Adherence to Ethical Standards in DoD-Supported Research," March 25, 2002.

Department of Defense Directive (DoDD) 6200.04, "Force Health Protection," October 9, 2004.

Department of Defense Directive (DoDD) 6490.2, "Comprehensive Health Surveillance," October 21, 2004.

Department of Defense Directive (DoDD) 6490.02E, "Comprehensive Health Surveillance," October 21, 2004.

Department of Defense Instruction (DoDI) 6490.3, "Implementation and Application of Joint Medical Surveillance for Deployments," August 7, 1997.

Department of Defense Instruction (DoDI) 1300.18, "Military Personnel Casualty Matters, Policies and Procedures," December 18, 2000.

Department of Defense Instruction (DoDI) 6025.19, "Individual Medical Readiness," January 3, 2006.

Department of Defense Instruction (DoDI) 6490.03, "Deployment Health," August 11, 2006.

Department of Defense Serum Repository, "Guidelines for Collecting, Maintaining, Requesting, and Using Specimens Stored in the Department of Defense Serum Repository," May 29, 2003.

Department of Defense Task Force on the Future of Military Health Care Final Report, December 20, 2007, p. 9. As of January 24, 2008:
http://www.dodfuturehealthcare.net/

Gillert, Douglas J., "Who Are You? DNA Registry Knows," American Forces Press Service, July 13, 1998. As of March 4, 2008:
http://www.defenselink.mil/news/newsarticle.aspx?id=41418

Hsu, H. W., Grady, G. F., Maguire, J. H., Weiblen, B. J., and Hoff, R., "Newborn Screening for Congenital Toxoplasma Infection: Five Years Experience in Massachusetts, USA," *Scand J Infect Dis Suppl*, Vol. 84, 1992, pp. 59–64.

Institute of Medicine, The National Academy of Sciences, "Interactions of Drugs, Biologics, and Chemicals in U.S. Military Forces," 1996.

Institute of Medicine, "Protecting Those Who Serve," National Academy Press, 2000, p. 2. As of February 20, 2009:
http://www.nap.edu/openbook.php?isbn=0309071895

Joint Chiefs of Staff (JCS), MCM-0006-002, 2002.

Joint Chiefs of Staff (JCS), MCM 0028-07, November 2007.

Mei, J. V., et al., "Use of Filter Paper for the Collection and Analysis of Human Whole Blood Specimens," *Journal of Nutrition*, Vol. 131, No. 5, May 2001, pp. 1631S–1636S.

Mitchella, B. L., et al., "Impact of Freeze-Thaw Cycles and Storage Time on Plasma Samples Used in Mass Spectrometry Based Biomarker Discovery," *Cancer Informatics*, Vol. 1, No. 1, 2005, pp. 98–104.

National Health and Nutrition Examination Survey (NHANES), Lab Manual, 2001.

National Health and Nutrition Examination Survey (NHANES). As of March 4, 2008:
http://www.faqs.org/nutrition/Met-Obe/National-Health-and-Nutrition-Examination-Survey-NHANES.html

National Heart, Lung, and Blood Institute (NHLBI), biorepository web site. As of November 2009:
https://biolincc.nhlbi.nih.gov/home

National Heart, Lung, and Blood Institute (NHLBI), *Biological Specimen Repository Catalog 2004.* As of March 4, 2008:
http://www.nhlbi.nih.gov/resources/medres/reposit/contents.htm

National Heart, Lung, and Blood Institute (NHLBI), *Limited Access Dataset Programs.* As of March 4, 2008:
http://www.nhlbi.nih.gov/resources/deca/default.htm

National Heart, Lung, and Blood Institute (NHLBI), *NHLBI Factbook, Fiscal Year 2006—By Section.* As of March 4, 2008:
http://www.nhlbi.nih.gov/about/factbook/toc.htm

National Science and Technology Council, Committee on International Science, Engineering, and Technology Working Group on Emerging and Re-emerging Infectious Diseases, "Infectious Diseases—A Global Threat," September 1995.

Navy Environmental Health Center. As of February 11, 2008:
http://www-nehc.med.navy.mil/

Office of the Assistant Secretary of Defense for Health Affairs (ASD(HA)), Memorandum, "The DoD HTLV-III Testing Program," December 5, 1985.

Office of the Assistant Secretary of Defense for Health Affairs (ASD(HA)), Memorandum, "Policy for Pre- and Post- Deployment Health Assessments and Blood," October 6, 1998.

Office of the Assistant Secretary of Defense for Health Affairs (ASD(HA)), Memorandum, "Tri-Service Reportable Events Document," November 6, 1998.

Office of the Assistant Secretary of Defense for Health Affairs (ASD(HA)), Memorandum, "Reportable Disease Database," November 9, 1998.

Office of the Assistant Secretary of Defense for Health Affairs (ASD(HA)), Memorandum, "Establishment of DoD Centers for Deployment Health," September 30, 1999.

Office of the Assistant Secretary of Defense for Health Affairs (ASD(HA)), "Concept of Operations Document," 1999.

Office of the Assistant Secretary of Defense for Health Affairs (ASD(HA)), Memorandum, "Automation of Pre- and Post-Deployment Health Assessment Forms," May 21, 2004.

Office of the Assistant Secretary of Defense for Health Affairs (ASD(HA)), Memorandum, "Requirements for Blood Samples Before and After Deployments," January 27, 2005.

Office of the Assistant Secretary of Defense for Health Affairs (ASD(HA)), Memorandum, "Policy for Pre- and Post-Deployment Serum Collection," March 14, 2006.

Office of the Under Secretary of Defense for Personnel and Readiness, Memorandum, "Enhanced Post-Deployment Health Assessments," April 22, 2003.

Presidential Decision Directive NSTC-7, "Emerging Infectious Diseases," 1996.

Public Law 105-85, National Defense Authorization Act for Fiscal Year 1998, Section 765, November 1997.

Public Law 105-261, National Defense Authorization Act for Fiscal Year 1999, October 1998.

Rai, A. J., et al., "HUPO Plasma Proteome Project Specimen Collection and Handling: Towards the Standardization of Parameters for Plasma Proteome Specimens," *Proteomics*, Vol. 5, No. 13, August 2005, pp. 3262–3277.

Rubertone, Mark V., MD MPH, and John F. Brundage, MD MPH, "The Defense Medical Surveillance System and the Department of Defense Serum Repository: Glimpses of the Future of Public Health Surveillance," *American Journal of Public Health*, Vol. 92, No. 12, December 2002.

Shafer, F. E., Lorey, F., Cunningham, G. C., Klumpp, C., Vichinsky, E., and Lubin, B., "Newborn Screening for Sickle Cell Disease: 4 Years of Experience from California's Newborn Screening Program," *J Pediatr Hematol Oncol*, Vol. 18, No. 1, 1996, pp. 36–41.

Steinberg, K., et al., "DNA Banking for Epidemiologic Studies: A Review of Current Practices," *Epidemiology*, Vol. 13, No. 3, 2002, pp. 246–254.

"UK Biobank Ethics and Governance Framework," Version 3.0, October 2007. As of September 4, 2009:
http://www.ukbiobank.ac.uk/docs/EGF20082.pdf

UK Biobank, "Improving the Health of Future Generations," homepage. As of March 4, 2008:
http://www.ukbiobank.ac.uk/

UK Biobank, "Sample Handling & Storage Subgroup Protocol and Recommendations," March 31, 2004.

UK Biobank, "UK Biobank: Protocol for a Large-Scale Prospective Epidemiological Resource," March 21, 2007.

U.S. Army Medical Research and Materiel Command, "Medical Research, Technology, and Materiel for the 21st Century Soldier, Sailor Airman, Marine" command brochure. As of May 14, 2008:
https://mrmc-www.army.mil/index.asp

U.S. Military HIV Research Program. As of March 4, 2008:
http://www.hivresearch.org/

Uttayamakul, S., et al., "Usage of Dried Blood Spots for Molecular Diagnosis and Monitoring HIV-1 Infection," *Journal of Virological Methods*, Vol. 128, No. 1–2, September 2005, pp. 128–134.

Zhang, Y.-H., and McCabe, E. R. B., "RNA Analysis from Newborn Screening Dried Blood Specimen," *Human Genetics*, Vol. 89, No. 3, May 1992, pp. 311–314.